'Coram Kidscape's work has shown us time and again that chronic bullying is traumatic – and must be recognised as such. We have seen the need for parents, carers and those working with children to have access to clear, accessible, trauma-informed guidance that gives them the confidence to respond to bullying sensitively and effectively. *Bullying and the Developing Brain* fills that gap with rigour, practical insight and, most importantly, hope that recovery is possible – and that informed adults, supportive relationships and coordinated systems can make all the difference.'

Kat Fuller, *Parent Support Manager, Coram Kidscape*

Bullying and the Developing Brain

This groundbreaking book shows how sustained bullying can affect children's developing brains and emotional wellbeing. Mental health educator Samantha Hill combines cutting-edge neuroscience with real-life stories to reveal bullying as a group-based social process – not just an individual incident. She translates complex research into practical guidance that addresses both individual children's needs and the peer cultures that allow bullying to persist.

The book provides clear, evidence-based strategies for recognising stress responses in children and supporting their recovery. With role-specific guidance for parents, educators and healthcare professionals, plus real-world case studies, Hill bridges neuroscience and everyday practice, while emphasising the brain's remarkable capacity to heal when children receive proper support.

Whether you're a parent noticing changes in your child, a teacher concerned about a quiet student, or a healthcare professional seeking to understand anxiety and school refusal, this book gives you the tools to respond effectively and help children recover their confidence and voice. It is essential reading for anyone committed to understanding and healing the impact of childhood bullying.

Samantha Hill is a lecturer, mental health educator and Interim Programme Lead at University College Birmingham. She teaches across health, mental health and nursing-related education, including the Student Nursing Associate programme, and has played a key role in developing and delivering the new BSc Mental Health and Wellbeing course. Her work focuses on the developmental, psychological and neurobiological impact of childhood bullying, with a particular interest in how trauma-informed approaches can support children, families, educators and health professionals.

Bullying and the Developing Brain

Understanding Trauma and Building Resilience

Samantha Hill

Routledge
Taylor & Francis Group
LONDON AND NEW YORK

Designed cover image: Getty images

First published 2027
by Routledge
4 Park Square, Milton Park, Abingdon, Oxon OX14 4RN

and by Routledge
605 Third Avenue, New York, NY 10158

Routledge is an imprint of the Taylor & Francis Group, an informa business

British Library Cataloguing-in-Publication Data
A catalogue record for this book is available from the British Library

ISBN: 9781041298816 (hbk)
ISBN: 9781041298809 (pbk)
ISBN: 9781003771777 (ebk)

DOI: 10.4324/9781003771777

Typeset in Optima
by Newgen Publishing UK

For every child who has felt unseen, unheard or unsafe, and for those still finding their way back to themselves.

Contents

Illustrations

Figures

Table

About the Author

Samantha Hill is a lecturer and mental health educator at University College Birmingham, where she teaches on the Student Nursing Associate programme. She holds an MSc in Mental Health Science and has a professional background in nursing education, mental health, trauma-informed practice and safeguarding. Her work focuses on the developmental, psychological and neurobiological impact of childhood bullying, with a particular interest in how trauma-informed approaches can support children, families, educators and health professionals. *Bullying and the Developing Brain: Understanding Trauma and Building Resilience* brings together neuroscience, mental health research, education, safeguarding and lived experience to challenge the idea that bullying is a harmless part of growing up.

Acknowledgements

This book would not have been possible without the support, encouragement and insight of many people.

I would like to thank my colleagues, students and professional networks, whose experiences and reflections have continually shaped my understanding of mental health, education, safeguarding and practice. Your openness, honesty and commitment to improving the lives of children and young people have been invaluable.

I am especially grateful to those working in education, healthcare, safeguarding and mental health roles, who continue to support children and young people affected by bullying. Much of this work is quiet, complex and often unseen, but it matters deeply.

Thank you to the researchers, practitioners and advocates whose work has informed and strengthened this book, particularly those advancing understanding of bullying, trauma, child development, neuroscience and recovery.

I would also like to thank my family and friends for their patience, encouragement and support throughout the writing process.

Finally, this book is for every child and young person who has experienced bullying and felt unheard, unsafe or alone. Your experiences matter. Your distress deserves to be taken seriously. And your recovery matters too.

Introduction

Why Bullying Is a Public Health Concern

Abstract

Bullying is often framed as a disciplinary issue within schools, yet growing evidence suggests that sustained peer victimisation may have significant implications for children's mental health, educational engagement and long-term wellbeing. This book approaches bullying as a social and developmental phenomenon rather than a series of isolated incidents. Drawing on international prevalence data, psychological research and emerging findings from developmental neuroscience, it examines how repeated exposure to peer aggression can affect stress regulation, identity formation and social belonging. The focus is primarily on children who are bullied and those who both bully others and experience victimisation themselves, while also acknowledging the complex pathways that lead some children to engage in bullying behaviour. By situating bullying within a public health framework, this book aims to support parents, educators and health professionals in understanding not only what bullying is, but why it matters across the lifespan.

In This Chapter

- What bullying is (and isn't), and why repetition and power imbalance matter
- Why bullying is a public health issue, not just a behavioural issue
- How bullying shows up across settings (schools, friendships, online spaces)
- Why some children are more exposed or more affected than others
- How to use this book in a practical, 'dip in and out' way

Why Bullying is a Public Health Concern

Bullying has frequently been described as an unfortunate but ordinary part of childhood. In many school settings it is addressed primarily as a behavioural problem requiring discipline or conflict resolution. While behavioural

DOI: 10.4324/9781003771777-1

accountability remains important, this framing alone does not capture the broader developmental implications of sustained peer victimisation. For some children, bullying is not a single disagreement or moment of conflict, but an ongoing social position within peer hierarchies. It is this chronic positioning, particularly when combined with power imbalance and repetition, that may carry developmental significance.

International data continue to show that bullying is widespread across educational systems. Global estimates from the United Nations Educational, Scientific and Cultural Organisation (UNESCO) indicate that approximately one in three young people report having experienced bullying during their schooling (UNESCO, 2019). In the United Kingdom, the Annual Bullying Survey 2020, drawing on the experiences of over 13 000 young people aged 12 to 18, reported that 25 percent had been bullied within the previous 12 months, representing a 25 percent increase compared with the previous year (Ditch the Label, 2020). The same report documented high levels of associated distress, with 44 percent reporting anxiety, 36 percent reporting depression, 33 percent reporting suicidal thoughts and 27 percent reporting self-harm following bullying experiences (Ditch the Label, 2020).

These figures do not imply that bullying inevitably causes severe psychological harm. Many children demonstrate resilience, supported by protective relationships, school culture and family stability. However, the consistency of associations between peer victimisation and mental health difficulties across studies suggests that bullying should not be regarded as trivial. Rather, it may represent a modifiable risk factor within a broader network of influences on child development.

Conceptual Clarification

Before positioning bullying as a public health issue, it is necessary to clarify what is meant by the term. Bullying is distinct from ordinary peer conflict. Conflict typically involves disagreement between individuals of relatively equal social power. Bullying, by contrast, involves three defining features: repetition, intention to harm, and an imbalance of power. That power imbalance may be physical, social, psychological or digital. It may derive from popularity, group status, perceived difference or structural inequalities embedded within wider society.

Bullying can take multiple forms. Physical aggression remains visible and often attracts adult intervention. However, research consistently shows that relational exclusion, verbal humiliation and rumour-spreading are among the most common forms of peer victimisation (Ditch the Label, 2020). In contemporary contexts, digital technologies have expanded the arenas in which such behaviour can occur. Online harassment, image-based abuse and social media exclusion may extend victimisation beyond school hours, reducing opportunities for respite.

Definitions explain what bullying is, but they do not fully explain why it persists. To understand persistence, it is necessary to consider peer group dynamics, social status and the role of bystanders. In practical terms, bullying often continues when peer groups reward or tolerate it, and it reduces when peer norms shift and help-seeking is made safe.

Bullying as Social Position and Group Process

Bullying should not be conceptualised solely as an 'event'. For some children, it represents a stable identity position within peer hierarchies. A child may become known as the one who is excluded, mocked or targeted. This social positioning can shape how others respond to them, how teachers interpret their behaviour and how they come to understand themselves. When this positioning becomes entrenched, the psychological impact may extend beyond immediate distress to influence identity formation and social expectations

Social network research indicates that bullying is often sustained through group processes rather than occurring as a simple exchange between two individuals. Peer norms, loyalty within friendship groups and fear of losing status can reinforce harmful behaviour. Bystanders therefore play a critical role. When peers remain silent or join in, bullying gains social strength. When peers offer support, challenge harmful behaviour or seek adult help, the dynamic can shift. Even a single act of prosocial intervention can signal that aggression is not endorsed by the group, and can help disrupt the pattern.

Scope of This Book

This book focuses primarily on children who are bullied and those who occupy the complex position of both bullying others and being bullied themselves, often referred to as bully-victims. These groups show higher levels of psychological distress and social vulnerability in multiple studies. While children who bully others are also considered, particularly in relation to developmental pathways and environmental influences, the central emphasis is on understanding the experiences and needs of those who are harmed by peer victimisation.

Throughout, person-first language is used. The terms 'children who are bullied' and 'children who bully' are preferred to fixed labels such as 'victims' or 'bullies'. This reflects an understanding that behaviour and experiences occur within contexts and do not define a child's identity permanently.

This book does not argue that all bullying experiences lead to trauma or long-term pathology. Nor does it suggest that bullying alone explains mental health outcomes. Rather, it examines how repeated peer victimisation can interact with individual vulnerability, family context, school environment and broader social structures to influence developmental trajectories.

Prevalence and International Context

Prevalence rates vary internationally due to differences in measurement tools, definitions and reporting cultures. The Ditch the Label Annual Bullying Survey 2020 reported high levels of self-reported bullying among young people in the United Kingdom (UK), including significant proportions experiencing relational and online abuse (Ditch the Label, 2020). The Anti-Bullying Alliance similarly reports that a substantial minority of young people in the UK experience bullying within a 12-month period (Anti-Bullying Alliance, 2020).

International organisations, including UNESCO and the World Health Organization, have recognised bullying as a global educational and health concern. UNESCO reports indicate that bullying affects a significant proportion of children worldwide, often linked to social inequalities and identity-based marginalisation (UNESCO, 2020). World Health Organisation (WHO) data situate bullying within broader frameworks of adolescent health and risk behaviour.

Patterns differ across regions. Cultural norms influence reporting. School systems vary in policy implementation. Nonetheless, the mechanisms of power imbalance, exclusion and social dominance are observable across contexts. Bullying is therefore both culturally situated and globally relevant.

Digital Environments and Changing Social Worlds

Children's social worlds have changed significantly over the past two decades. Digital communication has expanded opportunities for connection, but also for surveillance, comparison and harassment. The Annual Bullying Survey reported that 27 percent of those bullied experienced cyberbullying (Ditch the Label, 2020). Digital victimisation may involve persistent messaging, public humiliation, image-sharing or exclusion from online groups.

Digital environments differ from face-to-face contexts in several ways. Harmful content can be shared rapidly and widely. Anonymity may reduce empathy. Victimisation can occur at any time of day, reducing the possibility of safe spaces. However, digital platforms also provide opportunities for support, advocacy and connection. It is therefore important to avoid framing technology as inherently harmful. The focus instead should be on digital literacy, platform accountability and supportive adult engagement.

Identity-based Bullying and Intersectionality

Bullying does not occur in a social vacuum. Children are embedded within broader systems of inequality relating to race, disability, gender, sexuality, religion and socioeconomic status. Identity-based bullying targets aspects of a child's identity that are socially stigmatised or marginalised.

The Annual Bullying Survey found that perceived motives for bullying frequently related to appearance, interests, sexuality, disability and race (Ditch the Label, 2020). Children who identify as lesbian, gay, bisexual, transgender, and queer and questioning individuals plus (LGBTQ+), who have disabilities, or who belong to ethnic minority groups often report higher rates of victimisation in international studies. Intersectionality further complicates these experiences. A child who is both neurodivergent and from a minority ethnic background may experience layered vulnerabilities.

Recognising identity-based bullying is essential for two reasons. First, it highlights that peer aggression can reflect broader cultural attitudes and prejudices. Second, it underscores that prevention cannot rely solely on individual behaviour management. Whole-school cultures, representation, inclusive curricula and anti-discrimination policies play critical roles in shaping peer norms.

This book introduces identity-based bullying in this introduction and explores it in greater depth in Chapter 1.

Trauma Nuance, Stress, and What Evidence Can and Cannot Claim

The language of trauma is increasingly used in discussions of bullying. It is important, however, to apply this term carefully. Trauma refers to experiences that overwhelm an individual's capacity to cope, often involving threat, fear or loss of control. Not all bullying experiences meet this threshold. Many children encounter peer conflict that, while painful, does not result in enduring psychological injury.

Nevertheless, for some young people, sustained and severe bullying may produce trauma-like symptoms. These can include hypervigilance, avoidance, intrusive memories and negative self-beliefs. The Ditch the Label survey reported that 63 percent of those bullied described moderate to extreme impact on their mental health (Ditch the Label, 2020). These findings align with broader research linking peer victimisation to increased risk of anxiety disorders, depressive symptoms and self-harm.

Understanding stress responses does not require assuming damage or inevitability. The purpose of including stress and developmental science in this book is to explain why repeated social threat can feel overwhelming for some children, and why supportive environments can be protective. Developmental neuroscience provides a framework for understanding why sustained social threat may have psychological consequences. The stress response system, involving the hypothalamic–pituitary–adrenal axis and associated neural networks, plays a central role in regulating responses to perceived danger. Chronic activation of this system during childhood may influence emotional regulation and stress sensitivity. However, evidence in this field remains developing. Most studies identify associations rather than direct causal pathways. It is therefore more accurate to state that bullying can activate stress responses, and that repeated activation may influence development, rather than asserting that bullying deterministically reshapes the brain.

Protective factors must also be emphasised. Secure attachment relationships, supportive teachers, peer allies and effective school policies can buffer stress responses and reduce long-term impact. Public health approaches therefore focus not only on risk identification, but on strengthening protective environments.

Bidirectional Vulnerability and Developmental Pathways

Causality in bullying research is complex. Certain temperamental traits may increase vulnerability to being targeted. Behavioural inhibition, social communication differences, anxiety sensitivity or executive functioning challenges may shape peer interactions. Twin studies indicate moderate heritability in traits associated with victimisation and perpetration.

Bullying may exacerbate pre-existing vulnerabilities rather than create them *de novo*. Conversely, sustained victimisation may intensify anxiety, withdrawal or reactive aggression, contributing to bully-victim profiles. These children often demonstrate higher emotional dysregulation and complex relational patterns. Recognising bidirectionality supports more precise intervention. It shifts focus from blame towards understanding interaction between individual differences and social context.

Educational Impact

Bullying affects not only mental health but educational engagement. Children who are bullied report reduced concentration, school avoidance and diminished academic confidence. In the Ditch the Label survey, 18 percent reported truancy following bullying experiences (Ditch the Label, 2020). Reduced school attendance can compound disadvantage, particularly for children already facing socioeconomic challenges.

Teachers often face complex decisions when addressing bullying. Responses must balance accountability, safeguarding and restorative practice. When handled effectively, interventions can reduce recurrence and support recovery. When dismissed or minimised, harm may intensify. Public health framing emphasises that school climate is a modifiable determinant of wellbeing.

A Public Health Framework

Public health approaches seek to prevent harm at population level, while supporting those already affected. Applying this framework to bullying includes surveillance and data collection to understand prevalence and trends, primary prevention through inclusive school cultures and social and emotional learning, secondary prevention through early identification and targeted support, and tertiary intervention through psychological and educational support for those harmed.

Bullying is associated with increased risk of mental health difficulties in adolescence and adulthood. Longitudinal research suggests that children who experience chronic victimisation may show elevated risk of anxiety, depression and social difficulties later in life. While outcomes vary, the potential long-term burden justifies early prevention. From an economic perspective, untreated mental health problems carry significant societal cost through healthcare use, reduced productivity and intergenerational transmission of disadvantage. Prevention is therefore not only ethically important, but economically rational.

Hope, Plasticity and Recovery

Central to this book is recognition of resilience. Many children who experience bullying do not develop long-term difficulties. Protective relationships, inclusive school cultures and timely intervention can significantly alter trajectories. Neuroplasticity research suggests that supportive relational environments and therapeutic engagement can promote recovery of stress regulation and emotional functioning. Healing is rarely immediate and varies between individuals, yet possibility remains. Bullying is neither trivial nor destiny.

What This Book will do for Readers

This book is written for parents, educators and health professionals who want clearer understanding and practical insight. It brings together evidence from psychology, education and developmental science, and translates that evidence into a coherent framework for recognising harm early, responding safely and supporting recovery. The chapters that follow examine how bullying operates within peer cultures, how stress and belonging shape children's wellbeing, why some children are more vulnerable than others, and what adults can do to restore safety and resilience.

Key Takeaways

- Bullying is a repeated pattern of harm within a power imbalance, not a one-off conflict
- Bullying affects health, learning and long-term wellbeing, so a public health lens matters
- Impact varies; risk increases when bullying is chronic and support is absent

- Digital and identity-based bullying can increase intensity and reduce escape
- The most effective responses focus on safety, support and consistent adult action

References

Anti-Bullying Alliance (2020) *Prevalence and impact of bullying*. Available at: https://anti-bullyingalliance.org.uk/tools-information/all-about-bullying/prevalence-and-impact-bullying/prevalence-bullying (Accessed: 22 February 2026).

Ditch the Label (2020) *The annual bullying survey 2020*. Available at: www.ditchthelabel.org/research-report/The%20Annual%20Bullying%20Survey%202020 (Accessed: 22 February 2026).

UNESCO (2019) *Behind the numbers: Ending school violence and bullying*. Paris: UNESCO.

UNESCO (2020) *Tackling cyberbullying and other forms of online violence involving children and young people: Fact sheet*. Available at: https://unesdoc.unesco.org/ark:/48223/pf0000379486 (Accessed: 22 February 2026).

Part I

The Neuroscience of Bullying

Chapter 1

Rethinking Bullying

More Than an Argument Between Children

Abstract

Bullying is frequently minimised as a conflict between children, yet contemporary research demonstrates that it is a structured group process rooted in power imbalance and peer hierarchies. This chapter reframes bullying as a relational and systemic phenomenon rather than a series of isolated incidents. Drawing on social network research, longitudinal studies and national prevalence data, it explores why some children are repeatedly targeted, why others engage in bullying behaviour, and why a subgroup experiences both roles. Particular attention is given to identity-based victimisation, neurodevelopmental vulnerability, temperament and environmental stressors. By distinguishing between children who are bullied, children who bully, and children who are both bullied and bully others, this chapter establishes a foundation for developmentally informed and context-sensitive intervention. Understanding bullying as a group-based process is essential if adults are to respond effectively and prevent longer-term harm.

In This Chapter

- Why bullying is a group process shaped by power and status (not just 'kids falling out')
- Who is more likely to be targeted, and how vulnerability can be misunderstood
- Identity-based bullying (including racism, homophobia, ableism) and why it cuts deeper
- The difference between children who bully, children who are bullied, and those who are both
- What this means for prevention and early intervention

DOI: 10.4324/9781003771777-3

A Note on Language

Throughout this book, person-first language is used wherever possible: children who are bullied, children who bully, and children who are both bullied and bully others. Research literature often uses terms such as victim, perpetrator or bully-victim. While analytically useful, such labels can become fixed identities. A child who repeatedly hears that they are a bully may internalise that description. A child described solely as a victim may begin to see themselves as powerless. Language shapes expectation. By emphasising behaviour and experience rather than identity, the focus remains on development, accountability and change.

Rethinking Bullying: More Than an Argument Between Children

Bullying is often described as a falling out between pupils or a normal part of growing up. Such interpretations obscure the structural features that distinguish bullying from ordinary peer conflict. Conflict is typically situational and reciprocal. Bullying, by contrast, involves repeated harm enacted within a power imbalance. The imbalance may derive from physical strength, social status, group membership, digital reach or perceived popularity. What differentiates bullying from disagreement is not simply aggression, but repetition, hierarchy and the reduced capacity of the targeted child to defend themselves effectively.

When adults treat bullying as isolated misbehaviour, they risk responding only to the visible incident. A comment in a corridor, a rumour shared online, or exclusion from a game may appear minor when viewed in isolation. Yet, for the child repeatedly positioned at the bottom of a peer hierarchy, these events accumulate. Bullying is therefore best understood not as disconnected episodes, but as a relational pattern embedded within social systems.

Bullying as a Group-based Process

Research over the past two decades has reshaped understanding of bullying. Rather than viewing aggression as an exchange between two individuals, social network studies demonstrate that bullying is embedded within peer hierarchies. In every classroom, pupils occupy differing positions of influence. Some are socially central and widely recognised. Others are peripheral, with limited visibility or protection.

Children who bully often occupy relatively central or high-status positions. Their behaviour is not always impulsive. In certain contexts, it functions strategically to maintain dominance. Public humiliation, exclusion or subtle intimidation may signal rank within the group. Children who are bullied are more likely to occupy marginal roles, with fewer alliances and defenders. This structural imbalance reinforces power differentials and explains why patterns persist.

Bullying is rarely sustained solely by the actions of one child. It is maintained by the responses, silence or endorsement of the wider group. When classmates laugh, share humiliating content, or remain passive, aggressive behaviour is socially rewarded. When peers challenge harmful behaviour or seek adult support, the dynamic can shift. Even small acts of prosocial intervention can weaken the reinforcement that sustains bullying.

This perspective explains why responses focused exclusively on punishing the child who bullies frequently fail to produce lasting change. Unless peer norms and classroom culture are addressed, the hierarchy that sustains the behaviour remains intact.

Prevalence and Scale

National and international surveys consistently indicate that bullying remains widespread. In England, a substantial minority of pupils report repeated victimisation within a 12-month period. Rates are higher among pupils with special educational needs and disabilities, those experiencing socio-economic disadvantage, and those identifying as lesbian, gay, bisexual, transgender, and queer and questioning individuals plus (LGBTQ+) (Anti-Bullying Alliance, 2023).

Patterns vary across countries and age groups. Younger children more commonly report direct physical or verbal bullying. As pupils move into adolescence, relational and digital forms become more prominent. Although measurement differences influence estimates, consistent findings demonstrate that bullying is neither rare nor trivial. It is a common developmental stressor with implications for emotional wellbeing, academic engagement and longer-term mental health.

If bullying is widespread, the next question becomes why it persists around certain children more than others.

Why Some Children are Targeted

Asking why a particular child is bullied must never imply blame. Responsibility always lies with the child who engages in bullying behaviour and with the group that permits or reinforces it. However, understanding patterns of vulnerability enables earlier and more effective intervention.

In peer cultures where hierarchy is strong and difference is made socially visible, some children may be positioned as easier targets. Some are temperamentally cautious and avoid confrontation. In supportive contexts, these traits reflect thoughtfulness. In status-driven groups, however, hesitation can be misread as weakness. Others show heightened emotional reactivity. Visible distress can unintentionally reward provocation when peers gain attention or status from eliciting a reaction.

Some children experience difficulty interpreting social cues. Misunderstandings can accumulate over time and influence peer positioning. It is essential to emphasise that these differences do not cause bullying. Vulnerability emerges from the interaction between individual characteristics and the social environment, particularly the norms and behaviour that adults allow to develop.

This interactional view helps explain why the same child can thrive in one setting and struggle in another, and underpins the role of temperament and environmental sensitivity discussed next.

Temperament, Biology and Sensitivity to Social Threat

The suggestion that biology plays a role in bullying involvement can feel uncomfortable. It is therefore important to clarify what the evidence does and does not imply. Genetic influence does not mean inevitability. It indicates that children differ in baseline tendencies, and these differences interact with social environments over time.

Twin studies suggest moderate heritability for traits such as behavioural inhibition, impulsivity and emotional reactivity. These traits are also associated with bullying involvement. A child who is highly reactive to perceived rejection may respond defensively. A child with impulsive tendencies may act before considering the consequences. These patterns do not determine outcomes, but may influence how a child is perceived within peer hierarchies and how they respond under social pressure.

More recent polygenic research points to modest associations between genetic liability profiles linked to attention regulation, mood instability or behavioural dysregulation and risk of both peer victimisation and bullying behaviour. Effect sizes are small and predictive power is limited. Social context remains far more influential than genetic predisposition. However, these findings support a developmental model in which vulnerability reflects interaction rather than individual flaw (Schoeler et al., 2019).

A particularly useful framework is differential susceptibility. Some children appear more environmentally sensitive. In hostile contexts they experience greater distress. In supportive contexts they benefit more profoundly. Sensitivity therefore becomes a capacity that can magnify harm or amplify resilience, depending on adult scaffolding.

For parents and teachers, this often resonates with lived experience. One child appears able to brush off teasing. Another carries it deeply. This variation may reflect temperament, stress physiology and relational history. In that context, telling a distressed child to 'ignore it' may overlook a genuine stress response. Teaching coping skills, strengthening peer alliances and reducing exposure to hostile contexts is more effective.

Two mechanisms help explain how biology and environment co-shape peer experience. The first is gene–environment correlation. Children do not passively receive environments. Their tendencies can evoke responses from peers and adults. For example, a child with impulsive tendencies may interrupt frequently. Peers may respond with irritation. If irritation becomes exclusion, the child's social world narrows. Impulsivity does not cause bullying, but it may increase exposure to negative peer feedback and reduce access to protective friendships.

The second mechanism is stress reactivity. Some children show heightened physiological responses to social evaluation. Heart rate increases rapidly and cortisol response may be stronger. These children often experience embarrassment or rejection more intensely. In supportive environments, sensitivity can foster empathy and attunement. In hostile environments, it may magnify distress and reinforce vigilance.

This helps explain why two children can experience the same teasing episode and respond very differently. One appears to dismiss it. Another ruminates for days. The difference is not weakness; it is variation in sensitivity.

For practitioners, the implication is practical. Children who appear most reactive may require more structured protection, not dismissal. A child who 'overreacts' may be more biologically sensitive to social threat, particularly if previous environments have been unpredictable or unsafe. This does not reduce accountability for harmful behaviour. Rather, it refines intervention. A child who bullies impulsively may need emotional regulation coaching alongside clear behavioural boundaries. A child who withdraws may need scaffolding to rebuild peer alliances and restore a sense of safety within the group.

Biology shapes response. Environment shapes outcome. Protective relationships buffer stress activation, predictable school environments reduce uncertainty, and secure friendships provide social defence. Vulnerability and resilience are therefore relational processes, not fixed traits.

Family and Environmental Context

Children do not enter school as blank slates. Early relational experiences shape how they interpret social threat, and how quickly they expect rejection.

Consistent, emotionally responsive caregiving supports self-regulation and confidence in seeking help. Children raised in stable environments are often better equipped to form protective friendships and trust adults.

Children exposed to chronic stress, harsh discipline or persistent family conflict may enter peer environments with heightened vigilance. Some become defensive and reactive when they perceive rejection, others withdraw and anticipate criticism.

These patterns are not evidence of weak character. They are adaptive responses to environments that have felt unpredictable.

School climate also matters. Chaotic classrooms, unclear expectations and inconsistent adult responses create fertile ground for status competition. In contrast, classrooms that explicitly teach empathy, cooperation and inclusion reduce hierarchy-driven aggression.

Bullying therefore emerges from layered systems: temperament, family context, peer networks and institutional climate.

Identity-based Bullying and Neurodiversity

Identity-based bullying occurs when difference becomes a marker of social hierarchy. Children absorb cultural messages about race, gender, disability, sexuality and class. These messages shape peer norms long before adults intervene.

Children with special educational needs and disabilities consistently report higher rates of victimisation. Differences in communication, sensory processing, mobility or behaviour may draw attention in environments that prioritise conformity.

Neurodiversity and Bullying Risk

Neurodiversity describes natural variation in attention, sensory processing, communication and emotional regulation. Autism, attention-deficit/hyperactivity disorder (ADHD), dyspraxia and dyslexia reflect cognitive diversity rather than deficit. However, in environments that reward rapid social navigation and implicit rule-following, neurodivergent pupils can become more visible within peer hierarchies and are therefore more exposed to targeting.

Autistic children may interpret language literally, miss sarcasm or struggle to detect subtle exclusion. Direct communication may be misread by peers as rudeness or disinterest. Over time, repeated misunderstandings can contribute to marginalisation and reduced peer protection.

Sensory sensitivity adds further complexity. Noise, crowding and unexpected touch can overwhelm some pupils, particularly in corridors, dining halls and busy classrooms. Visible distress can then be exploited. Where peers identify predictable triggers, provocation can become patterned, with bullying embedded in the routines and spaces of school life.

When bullying is sustained and adult misunderstanding persists, some neurodivergent children internalise negative narratives about themselves. A child repeatedly labelled 'too sensitive' may suppress emotional expression. A child repeatedly removed from class for dysregulation may disengage academically. These responses are rarely fixed traits. They are often shaped by repeated experiences of social threat, correction and exclusion.

Exclusionary discipline disproportionately affects pupils with special educational needs and disabilities. Removal from mainstream spaces can reduce access to prosocial peer networks, increase isolation and reinforce low-status positioning. Without deliberate inclusion strategies, vulnerability can become entrenched.

Conversely, when neurodivergent pupils receive structured support, peer education and consistent adult advocacy, trajectories change. Protective peer alliances are more likely to form, regulation improves and academic engagement stabilises. The difference lies not in diagnosis, but in the environment.

Adult interpretation is pivotal. When shutdowns or meltdowns are framed as defiance rather than dysregulation, responses may become punitive, increasing both exposure and shame. Anti-bullying approaches therefore require adaptation and consistent implementation for pupils with special educational needs, rather than generic application.

Masking further complicates identification. Many neurodivergent pupils, particularly girls, camouflage differences to avoid rejection. They may appear socially competent in school while experiencing significant anxiety internally. Parents may then see exhaustion and distress at home that is not visible in the classroom. Without coordinated communication, bullying may remain hidden.

Neurodiversity also intersects with other identities. Neurodivergent pupils who are also from minority ethnic backgrounds or who identify as LGBTQ+ may face layered marginalisation, intensifying risk through compounding isolation and reduced access to defenders.

For clinicians, bullying should be considered when neurodivergent children present with anxiety, sleep disturbance, somatic complaints or school refusal, particularly during transitions. National data on bullying and online experiences among children in England and Wales reinforce the importance of routine enquiry about peer relationships and digital harassment in assessment contexts.

For schools, prevention requires explicit education about neurodiversity as human variation. Peer understanding reduces stigma. Structured supervision in high-risk spaces and staff training that distinguishes dysregulation from defiance can reduce escalation and prevent exclusionary responses from reinforcing vulnerability.

ADHD, Rejection Sensitivity and Online Risk

Children with ADHD may be disproportionately vulnerable in digital peer spaces because rapid, high-volume communication rewards fast responses and can escalate misunderstanding. Group chats and gaming environments can intensify impulsive exchanges, and reputational harm may be extended through screenshots, reposting and pile-on dynamics.

Rejection sensitivity can further amplify distress, particularly where micro-exclusions accumulate, for example being left on read, removed from group chats or mocked through memes. These patterns are easily missed by adults because they are relational rather than overt. Routine enquiry about online peer relationships should therefore be standard in school pastoral work and clinical assessment, particularly when neurodivergent pupils present with anxiety, sleep disturbance, somatic symptoms or school refusal.

This digital context is not a separate phenomenon from the school environment; it is an extension of peer hierarchy into a space where supervision is limited and harms can scale quickly.

Case Study: Bully-victim Pathway

Liam (pseudonym), aged 12, had a history of both being bullied and bullying others. In primary school, he was frequently teased for being small for his age. He struggled academically and often reacted strongly when mocked. In Year 7, his behaviour shifted. He began intimidating a younger pupil during break times.

Teachers initially viewed Liam as a troublemaker. He received detention and short-term exclusions. However, further exploration revealed a more complex picture.

Liam described feeling constantly on edge. He reported being pushed in corridors and excluded from online gaming groups. He said that targeting a younger pupil made him feel 'less weak'. His aggression functioned as protection against humiliation.

At home, Liam's parents were navigating financial strain and frequent conflict. Routine was inconsistent. Emotional support was limited, not through lack of care, but through exhaustion and stress.

Intervention required dual focus. Liam needed protection from peer victimisation and structured support to develop healthier responses. A pastoral mentor worked with him weekly to build emotional awareness and coping strategies. Staff increased supervision in identified hotspots. Restorative conversations addressed harm caused to the younger pupil while maintaining accountability.

Progress was gradual. There were setbacks. However, as peer alliances strengthened and adult responses became consistent, Liam's need to assert dominance reduced.

This case illustrates why simplistic labelling fails. Children who both bully and are bullied often require trauma-informed, developmentally sensitive approaches that balance protection with responsibility.

Case Study: Identity-based Targeting

Aisha (pseudonym), aged 14, wore a headscarf and had recently moved schools. Within weeks, she noticed classmates whispering and laughing during lessons. On social media, anonymous comments questioned whether she was 'oppressed' or 'allowed to have fun'.

Initially, Aisha minimised the incidents. Her attendance began to drop. She complained of stomach aches on school mornings. Teachers observed withdrawal but did not immediately connect it to peer hostility.

When a trusted staff member invited conversation, Aisha described feeling as though she 'did not belong anywhere'. The comments targeted not her personality but her identity.

The school response extended beyond sanctioning individuals. Staff reinforced anti-discrimination policies, reviewed supervision during transitions and incorporated inclusive dialogue into assemblies and classroom discussions. Aisha was offered a safe space to process her experience without being positioned as a spokesperson for her community.

Resolution was not immediate. Trust required time. However, visible adult leadership and peer support gradually strengthened her sense of safety.

This case demonstrates that identity-based bullying often operates subtly and requires proactive cultural leadership rather than reactive discipline alone.

Children Who Bully

Children who engage in bullying behaviour are often portrayed as inherently cruel.

For some, aggression functions as a strategy to secure or maintain social status. In environments where dominance is rewarded, bullying can confer influence. These children may be socially skilled and aware of peer dynamics.

For others, bullying reflects dysregulation. Exposure to harsh discipline, community violence or chronic stress may increase aggressive responses. Impulsivity, difficulty interpreting social cues or unresolved anger can shape behaviour.

Understanding these drivers does not excuse harm. Accountability remains essential. However, punishment without skill development often reinforces cycles of exclusion.

Effective intervention combines firm boundaries with emotional education, social skills development and consistent adult modelling.

Bully-victims: A Particularly Vulnerable Group

Children who both bully others and are bullied themselves often present the greatest challenge for adults, partly because their behaviour can obscure their vulnerability. They may appear disruptive, confrontational or defiant. Yet their aggression is frequently reactive, emerging in response to perceived threat, humiliation or social rejection.

Research indicates that this group often shows higher levels of emotional dysregulation than children who are solely bullied or solely bully others. Their social position can be unstable. They may not be accepted by dominant peers, yet their behaviour alienates potential allies. Shame and anger frequently coexist, and impulsive reactions can become a learned strategy for protection.

Longitudinal research suggests that bully-victims face elevated risk for later mental health difficulties compared to children who are solely bullied or solely bully others. Their aggression is frequently reactive rather than strategic.

Intervention for bully victims must therefore be layered. Safety from victimisation is essential. Simultaneously, these children require structured support to develop emotional regulation, conflict management and alternative responses to social threat. Restorative approaches can be effective when carefully facilitated and combined with consistent adult boundaries, rather than used as a substitute for safeguarding.

Developmental Sensitivity, Social Salience and Recovery

Adolescence is marked by heightened sensitivity to peer evaluation. During this period, social belonging becomes central to identity formation. Acceptance supports confidence and experimentation. Rejection can feel profoundly threatening.

Developmental neuroscience indicates that social reward systems become highly responsive during adolescence, while executive regulatory systems continue to mature into early adulthood (Crone and Dahl, 2012). This developmental asynchrony can intensify emotional reactions under stress and reduce regulatory capacity when a young person feels socially threatened.

In practical terms, repeated humiliation or exclusion may contribute to heightened vigilance, rumination and changes in sleep, concentration and mood. The key point is one of nuance. This evidence does not suggest that bullying deterministically damages the brain. Rather, repeated social threat during sensitive developmental windows may shape stress regulation patterns for some children, particularly when exposure is prolonged and support is limited.

Equally important is the capacity for recovery. When bullying stops and protective relationships are strengthened, stress responses often recalibrate. Young people are developmentally plastic. Supportive friendships, mentoring relationships and consistent adult reassurance can restore confidence and reduce anxiety over time.

For health professionals, this means screening early rather than waiting for symptoms to become entrenched. For teachers, it means responding to emerging marginalisation before it becomes chronic. For parents, it means taking subtle behavioural change seriously.

Bullying can influence developmental trajectory. It does not fix it permanently.

Risk, Bidirectionality and Complexity

The relationship between bullying and emotional difficulty is rarely one-directional. It is tempting to assume a simple causal pathway in which bullying leads to anxiety or depression. In many cases, victimisation does contribute to distress. However, developmental research increasingly demonstrates bidirectional processes.

Being bullied increases the likelihood of anxiety, low mood, school avoidance and anger. Repeated social threat can erode confidence and reduce a child's willingness to participate in classroom discussion or extracurricular activities.

Over time, withdrawal can reduce access to protective friendships, which may increase vulnerability to further exclusion (Nicola et al., 2024).

At the same time, some children who already experience anxiety, attention difficulties or behavioural dysregulation may be more likely to become targets. A child who hesitates socially, avoids eye contact or appears uncertain may be positioned as lower in status within certain peer hierarchies. A child who reacts intensely to teasing may unintentionally reinforce targeting behaviour (Salmivalli, 2010; Veenstra and Huitsing, 2021).

Longitudinal research is particularly helpful here. Studies following children over several years suggest that peer victimisation and emotional symptoms can influence one another over time. Early anxiety may increase the likelihood of later victimisation, and later victimisation may intensify anxiety. This reciprocal pattern means that effective intervention must address both peer dynamics and emotional wellbeing, rather than treating them as separate problems (Nicola et al., 2024).

For children who both bully and are bullied, trajectories can be especially complex. Reactive aggression may initially function as self-protection. However, it often leads to peer rejection, which increases isolation and can contribute to further aggression. Without interruption, this cycle can consolidate into more persistent behavioural difficulty (Salmivalli, 2010; Veenstra and Huitsing, 2021).

Importantly, outcomes are not fixed. The majority of children who experience bullying do not develop long-term psychiatric disorders. Protective relationships, timely adult intervention and stable school environments significantly reduce risk. However, when bullying is chronic, identity-based or combined with existing vulnerability, the likelihood of sustained distress increases (Wolke et al., 2013).

Understanding trajectory encourages early action. Waiting for symptoms to escalate can allow patterns to consolidate. Small behavioural shifts, such as reluctance to attend school, sudden irritability, sleep disturbance or somatic complaints, may signal relational stress long before formal mental health thresholds are met (Wolke et al., 2013).

For parents, this means noticing patterns rather than isolated incidents. For teachers, it means monitoring peer positioning across terms, not only responding to reported episodes. For health professionals, it means routinely considering peer relationships during assessment even when a child presents primarily with mood or physical symptoms (Wolke et al., 2013).

Bullying is not merely an event. It is a developmental context (Crone and Dahl, 2012).

Long-term Associations and Protective Factors

Longitudinal studies have identified associations between persistent childhood victimisation and later mental health difficulties, including anxiety and depressive symptoms, and in some cases reduced educational or occupational stability. These outcomes are probabilistic rather than deterministic, and pathways vary considerably (Wolke et al., 2013).

Protective relationships are consistently associated with better outcomes. The presence of even one stable, supportive adult can reduce risk. Secure friendships also buffer negative effects. School climate, family stability and community cohesion further shape trajectory and recovery (Wolke et al., 2013).

It is therefore misleading to present bullying as either harmless or inevitably damaging. Risk increases with duration, intensity, identity-based targeting and concurrent vulnerability. Protection increases with reliable relationships, early intervention and environments that reduce social threat (Wolke et al., 2013).

For bully-victims, the pattern can be more complex. Evidence suggests this group often shows higher emotional dysregulation across time. Their dual exposure, as both targeted and reactive, can amplify instability. This reinforces the importance of layered intervention that addresses safety and skill development simultaneously (Salmivalli, 2010; Veenstra and Huitsing, 2021).

Understanding trajectory supports proportionate response. Not every child who experiences bullying requires specialist mental health intervention. However, chronic or identity-based victimisation warrants structured support, monitoring and coordinated action across home and school (Wolke et al., 2013).

From Hierarchy to Ecology: How Prevention Works

If bullying is sustained by peer hierarchies, prevention must reshape the ecology in which those hierarchies operate (Salmivalli, 2010; Veenstra and Huitsing, 2021).

Large-scale systematic reviews demonstrate that school-based anti-bullying programmes can reduce both perpetration and victimisation, although effects are typically modest and vary by implementation quality. This is important. There is no single programme that eliminates bullying entirely. What works consistently are coherent systems (Bowes et al., 2024; Gaffney et al., 2021). Effective prevention tends to include:

- Clear behavioural expectations consistently reinforced by adults
- Structured supervision in identified hotspots
- Explicit teaching about empathy, bias and bystander responsibility
- Visible support for defending behaviour
- Early response to low-level exclusion before it escalates (Gaffney et al., 2021).

The common mechanism across successful approaches is norm change. When peer approval shifts from dominance to inclusion, aggression loses social currency (Salmivalli, 2010).

Teachers hold disproportionate influence in this process. Small signals matter. Which behaviours are praised, who is invited to participate, and how subtle 'jokes' are handled all contribute to peer norms. When adults respond promptly and proportionately, they communicate that humiliation is not rewarded (Salmivalli, 2010; Veenstra and Huitsing, 2021).

Whole-school consistency is critical. If one teacher ignores low-level exclusion while another addresses it firmly, hierarchies remain unstable. Inconsistent responses can reinforce the impression that bullying is negotiable (Gaffney et al., 2021).

For pupils with additional vulnerabilities, prevention must be adapted. Anti-bullying programmes designed for general populations may require modification for children with special educational needs, including simplified language, explicit rehearsal of defending skills and additional adult scaffolding (Badger et al., 2024; Gaffney et al., 2021).

Digital environments require equal attention. Cyberbullying often mirrors offline hierarchies but can extend humiliation beyond school hours. Teaching digital citizenship, establishing clear reporting routes and involving parents in online safety conversations can reduce risk (Office for National Statistics, 2024).

Prevention is therefore not an assembly once a year. It is an ongoing cultural practice.

International Framing: A Global Developmental Concern

Bullying is a global developmental concern. Cross-national surveys consistently identify peer victimisation across continents, although prevalence varies. Differences often reflect broader social structures, including inequality, anti-discrimination policy, digital regulation and school climate norms (Cosma et al., 2024).

Countries with strong inclusion policies and consistent behavioural frameworks tend to report lower levels of persistent victimisation, although cross-national differences reflect complex structural factors. This does not eliminate bullying, but it reduces structural reinforcement of hierarchy (World Health Organization Regional Office for Europe, 2024).

International framing matters for two reasons. First, it challenges the assumption that bullying is inevitable. Variation across countries demonstrates that norms and systems are influential. Second, it reinforces that bullying is not merely interpersonal; it is shaped by cultural messages about power and belonging. Children internalise what societies normalise (Salmivalli, 2010).

For health systems, recognising bullying as a public health issue supports routine enquiry and early identification. For education systems, it supports investment in whole-school approaches rather than isolated disciplinary responses.

Bullying is local in experience, but global in pattern.

Structural Inequality, Cultural Messaging and Compounding Risk

Bullying does not occur in a cultural vacuum. Peer hierarchies reflect broader social hierarchies. Children absorb messages about race, gender, disability, class and power long before they fully understand them. These messages shape which differences are stigmatised and which confer status (Salmivalli, 2010).

Socioeconomic disadvantage can influence bullying involvement through multiple pathways. Schools serving economically deprived communities often face higher staff turnover, larger class sizes and reduced access to pastoral resources. These structural pressures may weaken the consistency required to stabilise peer norms. At the same time, children experiencing material hardship may encounter elevated stress at home, influencing emotional regulation and social response patterns (Department for Education, 2025).

Identity-based bullying compounds risk because it attacks not only social position, but personal belonging. A child targeted for race, religion or sexuality experiences threat to their core identity rather than situational behaviour. Such experiences may contribute to chronic vigilance and reduced institutional trust if adults are perceived as dismissive or inconsistent.

Intersectionality intensifies exposure. A neurodivergent pupil from a minority ethnic background may experience marginalisation across multiple domains simultaneously. These risks do not simply add together. They interact. Isolation may increase because fewer peers share similar identities. Reluctance to report may increase if discrimination has previously been minimised (Department for Education, 2025).

For schools, this underscores the importance of cultural leadership rather than reactive sanctioning. Anti-bullying policy must align with anti-discrimination policy. Staff confidence in addressing racist, ableist or homophobic language reduces normalisation. Silence can inadvertently reinforce hierarchy.

Health professionals should recognise that identity-based bullying may present through somatic symptoms or anxiety without explicit disclosure. Routine enquiry about peer relationships, including identity-related targeting, can uncover stressors that would otherwise remain hidden.

Structural awareness does not remove personal agency. Children who bully remain accountable for behaviour. However, understanding context strengthens prevention. When schools promote inclusive norms, provide visible representation and reinforce belonging, the social currency of humiliation decreases (Salmivalli, 2010).

The aim is not to pathologise difference, but to create systems in which difference is protected.

Implementation Fidelity and Realistic Prevention

Research consistently shows that anti-bullying programmes are more effective when implemented with fidelity (Gaffney et al., 2021). However, real-world schools face competing priorities. Staff turnover, examination pressure and resource constraints can weaken sustained delivery.

Implementation fidelity involves more than following a manual. It requires leadership commitment, staff training and ongoing monitoring. Brief assemblies or poster campaigns are insufficient if peer norms remain unchanged in daily interactions.

- Explicit teaching about bystander responsibility
- Clear and consistent response to low-level exclusion
- Structured supervision in high-risk spaces
- Regular review of incident patterns
- Adaptation for pupils with additional needs

Whole-school coherence is more important than programme branding. Schools that align behaviour policy, safeguarding practice and inclusion frameworks demonstrate stronger reductions in persistent victimisation.

Parents also play a preventive role. Open conversations about online behaviour, modelling respectful disagreement and reinforcing empathy contribute to children's relational skill development.

Prevention is therefore ecological. It spans home, school and community.

Implications for Parents, Teachers and Health Professionals

Understanding bullying as a relational and systemic process leads to specific actions across home, school and health settings.

For parents, early indicators often include changes in sleep and appetite, school avoidance, unexplained physical symptoms, irritability or withdrawal. Supportive responses begin with calm, open questioning and the validation of emotions before problem solving. Recording patterns rather than isolated incidents can help schools respond proportionately and identify persistent peer dynamics.

For teachers, effective prevention includes the active supervision of high-risk spaces, a consistent response to low-level exclusion before it becomes entrenched, and the visible reinforcement of defending behaviour. Informal mapping of peer dynamics, including who is repeatedly marginalised and who holds influence, can help staff anticipate where risk is accumulating.

For health professionals, bullying should be considered when children present with anxiety, low mood, somatic complaints, sleep disturbance or school refusal. Direct but sensitive questions about peer relationships can reveal hidden stressors. Where concerns emerge, collaboration with families and schools can strengthen protective networks and reduce ongoing exposure.

Across roles, the most consistent protective factor is the same, reliable adult support that makes help-seeking safe.

Moving Beyond Simplistic Narratives

Several myths persist. One is that bullying builds resilience. While some young people develop coping skills, resilience emerges from support rather than harm.

Another misconception is that children who bully are simply 'bad'. As discussed, aggression often reflects status dynamics, stress or learned patterns. Addressing behaviour requires accountability combined with skill-building.

A further myth suggests that cyberbullying has replaced traditional bullying. Evidence indicates that digital platforms amplify existing peer hierarchies rather than create entirely new ones.

Replacing simplistic narratives with evidence-informed understanding enables adults to respond with clarity rather than reaction.

Prevention as Cultural Leadership

Effective prevention requires visible adult leadership. Policies alone do not reshape hierarchies. Daily modelling does.

Children observe how adults respond to subtle exclusion: a raised eyebrow at a sarcastic comment; a redirecting question that restores dignity; a public acknowledgement of inclusive behaviour. These micro-responses accumulate.

Prevention is also relational. Mapping peer dynamics informally across the year helps identify pupils who are repeatedly marginalised. Early conversation prevents entrenchment.

Programmes are most effective when implemented consistently across staff. Partial adoption reduces impact. Staff confidence in addressing identity-based language is particularly important. Avoidance can be interpreted as tolerance.

Importantly, prevention includes supporting children who bully. Clear boundaries, combined with emotional coaching, reduce recurrence. Punitive exclusion alone often reinforces status competition and does not teach alternative relational strategies.

Digital prevention must match offline effort. Clear reporting routes, consistent follow-up and parental partnership reduce amplification of harm.

Bullying thrives in silence and inconsistency. It weakens in clarity and coherence.

Conclusion

Bullying persists not because children are inherently cruel, but because social hierarchies, developmental sensitivity and environmental stress can converge. Some children are temperamentally more reactive. Some are marked by a visible difference in settings that punish difference. Some learn that aggression confers status. Others attempt to protect themselves by striking first.

Understanding bullying as a group-based phenomenon does not remove individual accountability. Rather, it broadens responsibility to include peer culture, institutional climate and adult leadership.

Adults hold the leverage. By shaping peer culture, modelling respect, responding consistently and protecting vulnerable pupils early they alter the relational ecosystem in which bullying thrives. Chapter 2 builds on this foundation by examining how repeated social stress interacts with physiological stress systems, and why safety and belonging are fundamental to resilience.

Key Takeaways

- Bullying is maintained by peer dynamics and adult blind spots, not just individual behaviour

- Some children face compounding vulnerability (identity, difference, neurodiversity, social position)
- Bully-victims often need the most joined-up support (safety + skills + context change)
- Prevention works best when schools create belonging, clear norms and consistent follow-through
- Adults matter most when responses are calm, predictable and repeated over time

References

Anti-Bullying Alliance (2023) *Bullying, school experiences and wellbeing: A picture of pupil experience in England 2023*. (Report; author listed as Martha Evans).

Badger, J.R., Nisar, A. and Hastings, R.P. (2024) 'School-based anti-bullying approaches for children and young people with special educational needs and disabilities: A systematic review and synthesis', *Journal of Research in Special Educational Needs*, 24(3), 742–757. https://doi.org/10.1111/1471-3802.12665.

Bowes, L., Babu, M., Badger, J.R., Broome, M.R., Cannings-John, R., Clarkson, S., Coulman, E., Edwards, R.T., Ford, T., Hastings, R.P., Hayes, R., Lugg-Widger, F., Owen-Jones, E., Patterson, P., Segrott, J., Sydenham, M., Townson, J., Watkins, R.C., Whiteley, H., Williams, M.E., Stand Together Team and Hutchings, J. (2024) 'The effects and costs of an anti-bullying program (KiVa) in UK primary schools: A multicenter cluster randomized controlled trial', *Psychological Medicine*, 54(15), 4362–4373.

Cosma, A., Molcho, M. and Pickett, W. (2024) *A focus on adolescent peer violence and bullying in Europe, central Asia and Canada: HBSC international report from the 2021/2022 survey*. Volume 2. Copenhagen: WHO Regional Office for Europe. Available at: www.hbsc.org/publications/reports/a-focus-on-adolescent-peer-violence-and-bullying-in-europe-central-asia-and-canada/. (Accessed: 22 February 2026).

Crone, E.A. and Dahl, R.E. (2012) 'Understanding adolescence as a period of social-affective engagement and goal flexibility', *Nature Reviews Neuroscience*, 13(9), 636–650. https://doi.org/10.1038/nrn3313.

Department for Education (2025) National behaviour survey report: 2024 to 2025 Academic year. *Research and Analysis*, 20 November 2025. Available at: www.gov.uk/government/publications/national-behaviour-survey-report-2024-to-2025-academic-year. (Accessed: 22 February 2026).

Gaffney, H., Ttofi, M.M. and Farrington, D.P. (2021) 'Effectiveness of school-based programs to reduce bullying perpetration and victimization: An updated systematic review and meta-analysis', *Campbell Systematic Reviews*, 17, e1143. https://doi.org/10.1002/cl2.1143.

Nicola, E., Mastroyannopoulou, K., Reeves, H. and Pass, L. (2024) 'Longitudinal associations between peer victimisation subtypes and children and adolescents' anxiety: A meta-analysis', *Aggression and Violent Behavior*, 79, 102013. https://doi.org/10.1016/j.avb.2024.102013.

Office for National Statistics (2024) Bullying and online experiences among children in England and Wales: Year ending March 2023. *Statistical Bulletin*. Available at: www.ons.gov.uk/peoplepopulationandcommunity/crimeandjustice/bulletins/bullyingandonlineexperiencesamongchildrenin englandandwales/yearendingmarch2023. (Accessed: 22 February 2026).

Salmivalli, C. (2010) 'Bullying and the peer group: A review', *Aggression and Violent Behavior*, 15(2), 112–120. https://doi.org/10.1016/j.avb.2009.08.007.

Schoeler, T., Choi, S.W., Dudbridge, F., Baldwin, J., Duncan, L., Cecil, C.M., Walton, E., Viding, E., McCrory, E. and Pingault, J.B. (2019) 'Multi-polygenic score approach to identifying individual vulnerabilities associated with the risk of exposure to bullying', *JAMA Psychiatry*, 76(7), 730–738. https://doi.org/10.1001/jamapsychiatry.2019.0310.

Veenstra, R. and Huitsing, G. (2021) Social network approaches to bullying and victimization. In Smith, P.K. and O'Higgins Norman, J. (eds) *The Wiley Blackwell handbook of bullying* (Volume 1, pp. 196–214). Hoboken, NJ: Wiley-Blackwell. https://doi.org/10.1002/9781118482650.ch11.

Wolke, D., Copeland, W.E., Angold, A. and Costello, E.J. (2013) 'Impact of bullying in childhood on adult health, wealth, crime and social outcomes', *Psychological Science*, 24(10), 1958–1970. https://doi.org/10.1177/0956797613481608.

World Health Organization Regional Office for Europe (2024) One in six school-aged children experiences cyberbullying, finds new WHO/Europe study. *News Release*, 27 March 2024. Available at: www.who.int/europe/news/item/27-03-2024-one-in-six-school-aged-children-experiences-cyberbullying--finds-new-who-europe-study. (Accessed: 22 February 2026).

Chapter 2

The Brain Under Stress

Abstract

Stress is a normal and helpful part of childhood, supporting learning, motivation and adaptation when it is short-lived and buffered by supportive relationships. Problems arise when stress becomes frequent, unpredictable and difficult to escape. For some children, repeated bullying creates these conditions and can keep the body's stress response activated for longer than intended. This chapter explains, in clear terms, how chronic stress can place strain on developing biological systems, including the brain networks involved in threat detection, learning, attention and self-control. It distinguishes between what research shows with strong confidence about toxic stress in childhood and what is still emerging about bullying-specific pathways. Rather than suggesting permanent damage, the chapter emphasises vulnerability and variability: children respond differently depending on timing, duration, support and recovery opportunities. It also highlights neuroplasticity and why safety, stability, sleep and relational protection can help stress systems rebalance.

In This Chapter

- The difference between manageable stress, chronic stress and toxic stress
- Why bullying can become biologically 'sticky' when it's repeated and inescapable
- How stress can affect sleep, learning, emotion and behaviour (and be misread)
- Key systems involved (HPA axis, amygdala, hippocampus, prefrontal cortex)
- What recovery-supporting environments look like in real life

DOI: 10.4324/9781003771777-4

Stress in Childhood: Helpful, Harmful and Overwhelming

Stress is a normal and necessary part of childhood. It helps children respond to challenges, stay alert and learn to adapt to new situations. Short-lived stress, such as feeling nervous before a test or during a difficult social interaction, can support learning and development. In these situations, the body activates its stress response and then returns to balance once the challenge has passed.

Difficulties arise when stress becomes frequent, unpredictable and hard to escape. For some children, repeated bullying creates exactly these conditions. When a child feels unsafe in their everyday social environment, particularly at school or online, their body may remain in a state of heightened alertness. Over time, this sustained stress can interfere with emotional regulation, learning, and physical health and wellbeing.

This chapter explains how stress affects the developing brain in clear and accessible terms. It does not suggest that bullying permanently damages the brain. Instead, it shows how chronic stress can place strain on biological systems that are still developing, while also highlighting the brain's capacity to recover when safety, stability and support are restored (McLaughlin et al., 2019; Gee et al., 2021).

Methodological Note: What We Know – and What Science is Still Uncovering

Research across child development, psychology and neuroscience shows clearly that chronic stress in childhood can affect the body's stress systems and the brain networks involved in emotion, attention, learning and physical health. Across many studies, chronic stress is linked to differences in cortisol patterns, a slower return to a calm state after threat, and changes in how brain regions coordinate during stress (McEwen, 2017; McLaughlin et al., 2019; Gee et al., 2021).

It is also important to be clear about what this evidence does and does not show. Peer victimisation is consistently associated with heightened stress responses, emotional distress, and difficulties with concentration and learning. However, research is still developing when it comes to identifying direct, long-term brain changes that can be attributed to bullying alone, and many findings in this area are correlational rather than causal (Wolke and Lereya, 2015; Arseneault, 2018).

For that reason, this chapter uses cautious, evidence-aligned language. Rather than implying that bullying permanently alters the brain, it reflects the current consensus that repeated stress can place strain on developing systems, particularly when experienced often or during sensitive stages of development (Lupien et al., 2018; Bethlehem et al., 2022). These patterns describe increased vulnerability rather than inevitable outcomes. Importantly, they remain responsive to protective factors: when stress reduces and children experience safety, stability and supportive relationships, stress-related patterns can ease and healthy development can continue (McLaughlin et al., 2019; Gee et al., 2021).

When Stress Becomes Toxic: Why Bullying can 'Stick'

When a child senses danger, whether that danger is physical or social, the body responds automatically. The brain activates the stress response system and releases hormones such as cortisol and adrenaline. Heart rate increases, attention sharpens and the body prepares to react. This response is designed to protect, and, in short bursts, it plays an important role in helping children cope with challenges.

Difficulties arise when this response is triggered too often. Children who experience repeated bullying may begin to expect harm, even when no immediate threat is present. Their bodies may remain on alert, scanning for danger and struggling to return to a calm state. Over time, this pattern can lead to what researchers describe as chronic stress, where the stress response is activated repeatedly without sufficient opportunity for recovery (Shonkoff et al., 2012; McEwen, 2017).

Chronic stress is particularly challenging during childhood because the systems that help children regulate emotions, attention and behaviour are still developing. When these systems are placed under ongoing strain, everyday functioning can become harder. Concentration may slip, emotions may feel overwhelming and physical symptoms, such as headaches or stomach aches, may appear.

Bullying can be a particularly powerful source of toxic stress because it is interpersonal, often repeated, and closely linked to social threat, humiliation or exclusion. These experiences carry extra weight during childhood and adolescence when peer relationships play a central role in emotional security and identity development. Research consistently shows that children who experience peer victimisation are at increased risk of stress-related emotional and behavioural difficulties, particularly when the bullying is persistent or occurs across multiple settings (Arseneault, 2018).

Social Threat Circuitry: Why Bullying Feels Biologically Urgent

Bullying is stressful not only because it is unpleasant, but because it signals social threat. For children and adolescents, belonging is tightly linked to safety, identity and daily functioning. Social exclusion, humiliation, and public ridicule can therefore trigger the stress response in ways that feel immediate and intense.

When social threat is repeated, the brain and body can become more prepared for it. A child who has been targeted may begin to scan their environment for cues that something is about to happen: the look that precedes laughter, the group forming in the corridor, the phone notification that signals another message. This is not overreacting. It is a nervous system adapting to an environment that has become unpredictable.

Research in this area points to changes in the way young people process social evaluation, rejection and exclusion, with some studies finding heightened responsivity during exclusion tasks and greater activation in brain systems involved in monitoring social danger. These findings fit with a stress-based model of peer victimisation, where repeated experiences of exclusion can heighten vigilance and make it harder to feel safe, even when no immediate bullying is occurring (Ke et al., 2022).

This also helps explain why bullying can affect children across settings. Once a child has learned that peers are unsafe, the body may not simply 'switch off' at the classroom door. A child may appear distracted, tense or withdrawn because their attention has been pulled towards monitoring the social environment. For some children, this can look like anxiety. For others, it may show up as irritability or anger, particularly when they feel cornered or repeatedly embarrassed.

Importantly, this pattern is not permanent or inevitable. It is best understood as an adaptive response to threat: the brain invests resources in detecting danger because the environment has taught it that danger is likely. When the environment becomes safer, when adults intervene effectively, and when peer relationships become more predictable and supportive, these heightened patterns can settle. This is one reason why whole-school approaches and consistent adult response matter so much: safety is not only psychological. Over time, it becomes biological.

The Developing Brain: Why Timing Matters

The human brain continues to grow and change from early childhood into early adulthood. While the most visible stages of development occur in childhood and adolescence, research now shows that important processes such as refining connections between brain cells, strengthening communication pathways, and improving coordination between different brain areas continue well into a person's twenties and early thirties. These later changes are particularly noticeable in areas involved in planning, emotional control and complex thinking (Arain et al., 2013; Tamnes et al., 2017; Bethlehem et al., 2022).

Because brain development is ongoing for such a long period, children and young people remain sensitive to their environments. The systems that help manage emotions, regulate behaviour and process social information are still taking shape. Stressful experiences during these stages can therefore have a stronger impact, especially when stress is repeated, unpredictable or involves social threat. This does not mean that stress causes permanent damage. Instead, it can influence the direction development takes, particularly in areas linked to emotional regulation and self-control (McLaughlin et al., 2019; Gee et al., 2021).

Adolescence is a particularly sensitive time, but it should not be viewed as a period of inevitable vulnerability. During these years, young people become more aware of how they are seen by others, peer relationships take on greater importance, and the parts of the brain that support judgement and emotional control are still maturing. Research using modern brain imaging methods suggests that stress during adolescence can temporarily shift how the brain balances systems involved in control and threat detection. These changes often reflect differences in how brain networks work together, rather than permanent structural change (Moseley et al., 2022; Moseley et al., 2024).

Sleep also plays an essential role in this process. Biological changes during puberty and early adulthood can naturally affect sleep patterns, and stress can further disrupt sleep. Poor or irregular sleep has been linked to increased emotional reactivity and a reduced ability to manage stress, partly because tired brains struggle to regulate emotions and attention. Emerging research suggests that disrupted sleep may intensify the effects of stress by reducing the brain's capacity to settle and increasing sensitivity to perceived threat (Short et al., 2023; Gregory et al., 2024).

Taken together, this evidence highlights that brain development is a gradual and flexible process that continues well beyond adolescence. Importantly, it also shows that the brain remains capable of adjustment and recovery. When stress is reduced and children or young people experience stable, supportive relationships, stress-sensitive systems can rebalance. This ongoing capacity for change underlines the importance of timely support at all stages of development, not only in early childhood.

Sleep, Circadian Rhythm and Recovery: Why Nights Matter as Much as School Days

Sleep is one of the brain's most powerful regulators of stress. During sleep, the brain consolidates learning, processes emotion and supports the recovery of systems that have been activated by threat. When sleep is disrupted, stress becomes harder to manage, emotions become easier to trigger, and attention and memory can suffer.

Adolescence adds another layer. Puberty naturally shifts the body clock later, meaning many teenagers are biologically primed to feel sleepy later and wake later. This shift does not reflect laziness or poor routines. It is a developmental change. However, early school start times, academic pressure and social demands often work against it, increasing the likelihood of sleep debt. When bullying is added to this mix, recovery becomes even harder.

Children who feel unsafe often struggle to settle. They may replay events, anticipate what will happen tomorrow, or remain on alert for messages. This matters because the stress system does not only respond to what is happening now; it also responds to anticipated threat. If a child expects humiliation or exclusion the next day, their body may remain partially mobilised, even at night. Over time, this can contribute to the pattern many adults observe: difficulty falling asleep, restless sleep, early waking, nightmares and fatigue.

Sleep disruption is also one of the ways bullying can 'spill over' into daytime functioning. Tired brains are less efficient at regulation. Emotional reactions become stronger, concentration is harder to sustain, and minor social cues can feel more threatening. In practical terms, this can make school feel even less manageable, particularly for children already trying to navigate a hostile peer environment.

Digital life can intensify this cycle. Bullying no longer reliably ends when a child leaves school. Online harassment, exclusion from group chats, the threat of screenshots and constant social comparison can extend social threat into the evening. A recent review by Orben and colleagues highlights that the mental health effects of social media are mixed and not uniform, but it also identifies plausible mechanisms by which digital affordances can amplify adolescent vulnerability: heightened sensitivity to social feedback, social comparison, exclusion experiences and stress sensitivity during a developmental window when peer evaluation carries particular weight (Orben et al., 2024).

This does not mean that social media 'causes' stress responses in a simple way. The evidence is still developing, and many findings are inconsistent. However, the mechanism-based explanation is useful clinically and educationally: if a child is repeatedly exposed to social evaluation and exclusion cues at night, their nervous system may struggle to downshift, and sleep may be disrupted as a result. Orben and colleagues note that research on stress biology in relation to social media is still inconclusive, in part because cortisol varies across the day and is difficult to measure reliably (Orben et al., 2024).

For practice, the key point is this: sleep is not an add-on. It is part of the stress system. Supporting sleep can be a meaningful part of recovery. This might include predictable evening routines, limits on exposure to stressful online spaces before bed, calming wind-down activities, and addressing the underlying fear by ensuring bullying is taken seriously and is actively reduced. When safety improves, sleep often improves. When sleep improves, the brain becomes better able to regulate stress and re-engage with learning.

Key Systems Under Strain

The Amygdala: The Brain's Alarm System

The amygdala forms part of the brain's early warning system. It helps us notice danger and respond quickly to potential threats. When a child feels unsafe, whether because of physical danger or social stress, the amygdala becomes active and signals the body to prepare for action.

Research suggests that repeated social stress, including ongoing bullying, is associated with increased sensitivity in threat-detection systems. This means the brain may become quicker to register potential threat, even in situations that are ambiguous rather than objectively dangerous. Neuroimaging studies have found that some children exposed to chronic stress show higher amygdala reactivity, and some studies report differences in amygdala volume during childhood (Figure 2.1) (Teicher et al., 2016; McLaughlin et al., 2019; Ke et al., 2022).

Where differences in volume are reported, they are not best understood as 'damage'. Rather, they are often interpreted as an experience-related adaptation: when a child is repeatedly exposed to threat, the brain may allocate more resources to systems that support vigilance and the rapid detection of danger. Outcomes vary widely and are shaped by factors such as the duration and timing of stress, and whether the child has access to consistent, supportive relationships.

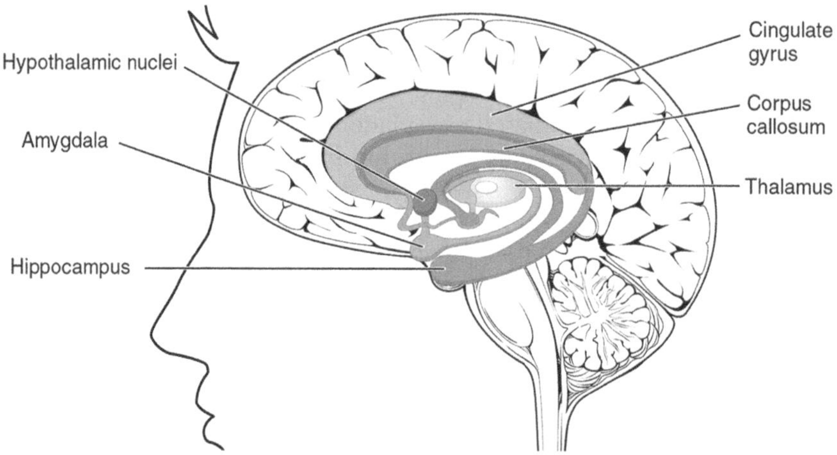

Figure 2.1 **Limbic system stress regions.** The limbic system and key structures involved in emotion and stress. Key regions include the amygdala, hippocampus, hypothalamus, thalamus, cingulate gyrus and corpus callosum, which contribute to emotional processing and physiological stress responses.

Source: OpenStax College (2013), CC BY 3.0.

When the amygdala remains highly sensitive, children may stay on alert even in safe environments. This can contribute to anxiety, avoidance of social situations, or strong emotional reactions to minor challenges. Heightened threat sensitivity has also been linked to disrupted sleep, which can further affect emotional regulation, attention and learning (Vaillancourt et al., 2013; McLaughlin et al., 2019).

The Hippocampus: Learning and Memory

The hippocampus is a brain structure that plays a crucial role in learning, memory and concentration. It helps children absorb new information, store it and recall it later. This system tends to work best when a child feels calm and safe.

The hippocampus is particularly sensitive to stress because it contains many receptors for stress hormones such as cortisol. When stress levels remain high for prolonged periods, these hormones can disrupt the hippocampus' usual functioning. Research consistently shows that long-lasting stress during childhood is associated with differences in hippocampal functioning, particularly when stress is repeated and hard to escape (Lupien et al., 2018; McLaughlin et al., 2019).

Neuroimaging and longitudinal studies in the broader stress literature suggest that some children and adolescents exposed to chronic stress show smaller hippocampal volumes compared with their peers who are not exposed to ongoing stress, often alongside difficulties with attention, working memory and retaining new information (Ke et al., 2022; Girotti et al., 2024). Importantly, these findings do not indicate 'brain damage' or the straightforward loss of brain cells. They are better understood as stress-related differences in how neural tissue develops and how connections are strengthened over time (Figure 2.2).

When the hippocampus is under strain, learning can become more difficult. Children may struggle to concentrate, forget instructions or find it harder to remember what they have learned in class. This can look like inattention or academic disengagement, but it often reflects the impact of stress on learning systems rather than a lack of effort or ability.

Some studies link experiences of bullying and peer victimisation with stress-related difficulties in memory and concentration. Rather than suggesting that bullying directly causes the hippocampus to shrink, current evidence supports the view that repeated social stress can reduce the brain's capacity to support learning while stress levels remain high (Ke et al., 2022; Menken et al., 2023). These effects are best understood as increased vulnerability rather than fixed outcomes.

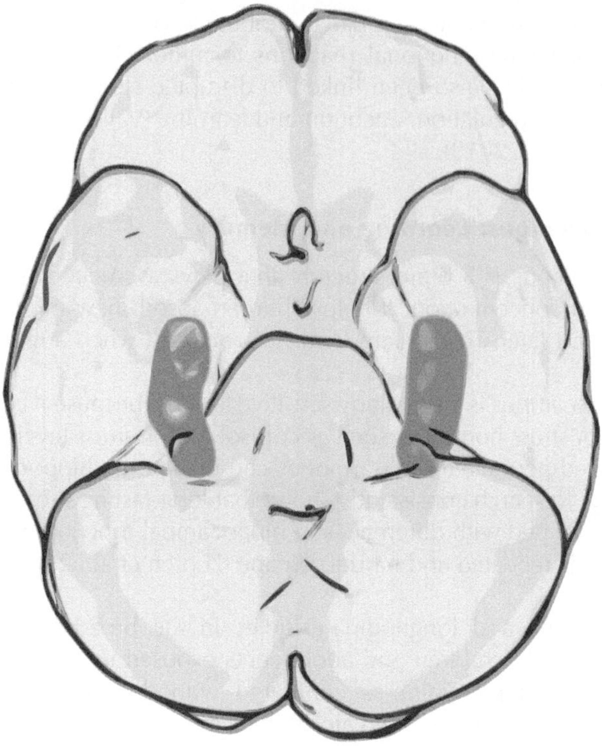

Figure 2.2 **The location of the hippocampus in the human brain.** The highlighted areas show the approximate position of the hippocampi within the temporal lobes. The hippocampus supports learning, memory formation and contextual processing, and is sensitive to prolonged stress exposure.

Source: Washington Irving (2020) *Hippocampus.svg*. Wikimedia Commons. Public domain, CC0 1.0.

Crucially, hippocampal functioning shows a strong capacity for recovery. Research suggests that, when stress is reduced and children experience predictable routines, emotional support and relational safety, learning and memory processes can improve over time (Lupien et al., 2018; Shonkoff et al., 2021). This highlights the importance of supportive environments in restoring a child's ability to engage, concentrate and learn.

The Prefrontal Cortex: Self-control and Problem-solving

The prefrontal cortex helps children pause, think, plan and manage emotions. It supports attention, decision-making, impulse control and problem-solving.

These abilities develop gradually and depend on stable communication between the prefrontal cortex and other brain systems.

Stress can interfere with how efficiently this system operates. Research shows that prolonged stress, particularly during childhood and adolescence, can reduce the effectiveness of prefrontal regulation. This does not mean the prefrontal cortex stops working or is damaged. Rather, it may become less able to manage emotions and behaviour while stress levels remain high (Arnsten, 2015; Arnsten et al., 2023).

Recent brain imaging studies suggest that stress affects how networks work together, rather than impacting a single brain region in isolation. Research by Moseley and colleagues indicates that adolescents exposed to ongoing stress may show weaker coordination within networks involved in planning and self-control, alongside a stronger influence from systems involved in threat detection and emotional salience (Moseley et al., 2022; Moseley et al., 2024). In practical terms, this can make it harder for young people to stay calm, think clearly and regulate their responses under pressure (Figure 2.3).

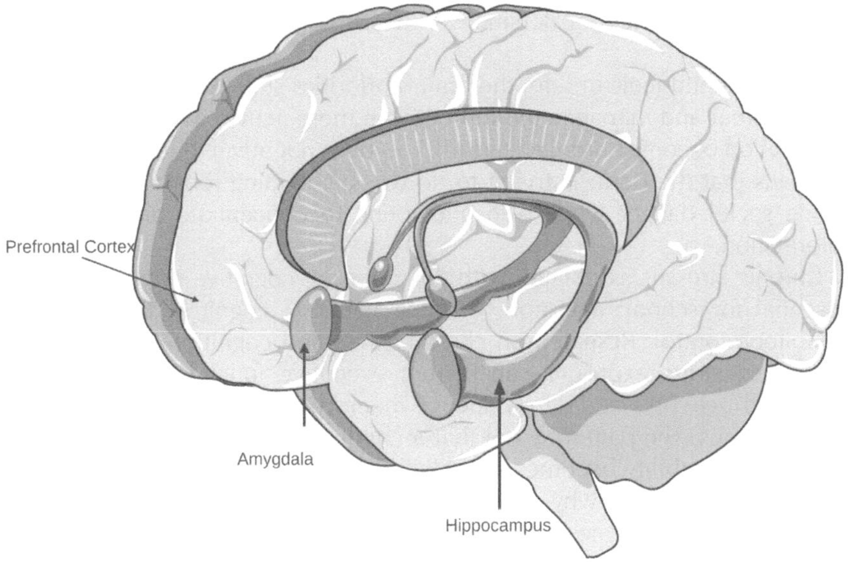

Figure 2.3 **Brain systems involved in stress regulation.** The prefrontal cortex supports planning, inhibition and emotion regulation; the amygdala detects potential threat; and the hippocampus supports memory and contextual processing. Under repeated stress, threat-detection systems may become more reactive, while regulatory and learning systems may work less efficiently. Adapted from Servier Medical Art, licensed under CC BY 4.0.

Source: Image provided by Servier Medical Art, https://smart.servier.com, licensed under CC BY 4.0, https://creativecommons.org/licenses/by/4.0/

When stress is repeated, the brain may prioritise rapid emotional reactions over thoughtful decision-making. As a result, children may act impulsively, struggle to concentrate, or experience emotional outbursts or withdrawal. These behaviours reflect reduced regulatory capacity during periods of stress, rather than deliberate defiance or poor character.

Importantly, these effects are not fixed. When stress reduces and children experience consistent support, safety and predictable routines, prefrontal regulation can strengthen again. This reinforces the importance of responding to stress-related behaviour with understanding and support, rather than punishment, and underlines the brain's capacity to recover as circumstances change.

Cognition Under Stress: Why Bullied Children may Struggle to Learn Even When They are Capable

Teachers often notice changes in learning before they hear about bullying. A child who previously engaged well may begin to drift, forget instructions, struggle to start tasks, or appear 'switched off'. These changes can be misinterpreted as laziness or defiance. A stress-informed view offers a different explanation.

When a child feels unsafe, the brain's priorities shift. Systems designed to detect threat and manage emotion become more active, while learning and exploration become harder to sustain. This does not mean that learning stops. It means that the brain is trying to do two demanding jobs at once: monitoring social danger while also attempting to concentrate and remember information.

Chronic stress is associated with difficulties in cognitive domains that are essential for school: attention, working memory, cognitive flexibility and inhibitory control. Research on chronic stress and cognition describes how prolonged stress exposure can disrupt executive functions supported by prefrontal networks and can influence memory processes supported by the hippocampus. The pattern is not that a child suddenly loses ability, but that access to that ability becomes less reliable under sustained strain.

This is one reason why bullying can lead to inconsistent performance. A child may appear fine in one lesson and then unravel in another, particularly if the social context changes (for example, group work with certain peers, unstructured transitions, or times of day when supervision is limited). For adolescents, sleep disruption can further reduce executive function and emotion regulation capacity, making concentration and impulse control harder precisely when academic demands increase.

Emerging longitudinal work strengthens this picture by linking bullying victimisation to later differences in cognitive performance and brain development trajectories. Menken and colleagues used data from the ABCD study and reported poorer cognitive performance in bullied children over time, alongside differences in brain morphometry, with some neural measures partially mediating associations with cognition. The authors also highlight limitations, including bullying measurement and the need for longer follow-up, which is consistent with a cautious interpretation: these findings suggest meaningful associations and plausible pathways, not deterministic damage (Menken et al., 2023).

For practice in schools, this helps reframe behaviour and learning difficulties as potential signals of stress exposure. Helpful responses include reducing uncertainty, increasing predictable routines, offering safe access to adults and providing options that reduce social threat during learning (for example, careful grouping, structured transitions and choices that preserve dignity). These adjustments do not replace anti-bullying intervention. They support the child's learning while the wider safeguarding work is being done.

For health professionals, this section also helps explain why bullying-related stress can present as 'attention problems', 'school refusal', or 'behavioural difficulties'. It supports careful assessment: what looks like inattentiveness may be vigilance; what looks like avoidance may be threat anticipation; what looks like impulsivity may be reduced regulatory capacity under chronic stress.

The HPA Axis: Stress on Repeat

The body has a system that helps regulate how it responds to stress. This system controls the release of stress hormones, including cortisol, and supports a return to balance once a threat has passed. In healthy circumstances, it switches on when needed and then switches off again.

For children exposed to repeated bullying or ongoing peer victimisation, this system can become overworked. Research shows that some children develop heightened stress responses, while others show a dampened or 'blunted' response over time. Both patterns reflect difficulty regulating stress, rather than resilience or weakness (Miller et al., 2011; Vaillancourt et al., 2013).

When the stress system is repeatedly activated, children may experience a range of physical symptoms. These can include headaches, stomach aches, fatigue, sleep problems and increased vulnerability to illness. Such symptoms are commonly reported by children under chronic stress and reflect sustained strain on the body's regulatory systems.

These responses are real and measurable. They should not be dismissed as exaggeration, attention-seeking or avoidance. Instead, they signal that a child has been under prolonged stress and needs support. Recognising this helps adults respond with understanding, appropriate care and early intervention, rather than disbelief or punishment.

From Stress Response to Allostatic Load: When the Body Carries Stress Over Time

The stress response is designed to protect. In short bursts, it helps children react quickly, focus attention and mobilise energy. The problem is not the stress response itself. The problem is when a child has to use it repeatedly, with little opportunity to recover. Over time, the body can begin to show signs of what researchers describe as allostatic load: the cumulative 'wear and tear' of repeated activation across multiple systems.

For children who experience ongoing bullying, the body may not only respond during the bullying event. It may also respond during anticipation ('Will it happen again today?'), during avoidance ('I'll take a longer route to class.'), and during social monitoring ('Are they laughing at me?'). This repeated activation can affect sleep, appetite, headaches, stomach aches, immune functioning and mood. These physical symptoms are not imagined. They are part of the body's attempt to adapt to persistent stress.

Over time, some children show heightened stress responses, while others show dampened responses, with the stress system becoming less reactive after prolonged strain. Both patterns can reflect a system that is struggling to regulate effectively, rather than a sign that a child is 'strong' or 'weak'. This fits with the broader stress literature and with evidence reviewed in the existing section on the HPA axis (Miller et al., 2011; Vaillancourt et al., 2013).

One reason this matters for health professionals is that bullying is increasingly recognised as a risk factor for later mental and physical health difficulties, including pathways involving inflammatory and metabolic processes. The background research summary notes that chronic stress related to bullying is discussed in relation to neuroendocrine, inflammatory and metabolic functioning, and that bully-victims often show the highest overall risk profile (Wolke et al., 2013; Takizawa et al., 2014; Wolke and Lereya, 2015; Suglia et al., 2021).

It is important to frame this carefully. These findings do not mean that bullying inevitably leads to long-term disease. They indicate that repeated social stress can become biologically embedded over time, particularly when it coincides with other adversities, limited support or ongoing exposure across settings. For some young people, the consequences may be primarily emotional and behavioural; for others, physical symptoms may dominate; for many, the impact may be mild or temporary when the bullying is stopped and support is restored.

From a practice perspective, the concept of allostatic load helps adults respond differently to children who present with vague or recurring physical complaints. Rather than assuming avoidance, attention-seeking or misbehaviour, adults can consider whether the child's body is carrying prolonged stress. This shifts the response towards safeguarding, reducing ongoing harm and restoring predictable safety.

Finally, allostatic load provides a bridge to hope. The body is plastic, as well as vulnerable. When stress reduces and children experience stability, sleep improves, supportive relationships increase and routines become more predictable, stress-related strain can ease. For many children, improvement is not immediate, but it is possible, particularly when adults respond early and consistently.

What Brain Imaging Can – and Cannot Yet – Tell Us about Bullying

Over the past decade, researchers have increasingly used brain imaging methods to explore whether peer victimisation is associated with differences in brain structure or function. This work is sometimes described in simplified ways in the media, but the research itself is more careful. Brain imaging does not tell us that bullying 'damages' the brain, and it does not allow us to point to a single, bullying-specific signature. What it can do is help us understand how repeated social stress may be linked to patterns in brain systems involved in threat detection, social evaluation, learning and regulation.

A systematic review by Ke and colleagues examined studies published between 2000 and 2021 that measured peer victimisation (including bullying and cyberbullying) and assessed structural or functional brain outcomes in young people up to the age of 25. Across 26 studies, the overall picture was consistent with stress and social-threat models: victimisation exposure was linked with differences in activation and connectivity in networks involved in social pain and exclusion, threat and salience detection, reward processing and emotion regulation. At the same time, the review highlighted an important limitation: many studies were cross-sectional and varied in how victimisation was measured, making it difficult to draw firm causal conclusions (Ke et al., 2022).

Several studies included in the review used experimental tasks designed to simulate exclusion or rejection. These tasks often activate brain systems linked to the distress of social rejection and the monitoring of threat or salience. In some studies, young people with histories of peer victimisation showed heightened reactivity during social exclusion tasks. In everyday terms, this fits with what many children and adolescents describe: when a peer environment has repeatedly been unsafe, signs of exclusion can feel especially intense, and the body may respond as though rejection is a serious threat.

It is important, however, not to overinterpret what this means. A stronger response to exclusion cues does not imply that a child is 'broken' or that their brain has been permanently changed. It may reflect an adaptive response to experience: the brain becomes quicker to register cues that have previously signalled harm. In supportive contexts, where social safety is restored and peer interactions become more predictable, these heightened patterns may ease.

Ke and colleagues also summarised studies involving brain regions commonly discussed in relation to threat sensitivity, including the amygdala and connected limbic systems. Some studies reported heightened activation during tasks involving negative social feedback, emotional faces or exclusion. Other studies found mixed or non-significant effects. Overall, the review supports cautious phrasing: peer victimisation is associated, in some samples and under certain conditions, with differences in how the brain responds to social threat or emotional cues, but the findings are not uniform across all studies or all children (Ke et al., 2022).

This variability matters for practice. It reminds us that there is no single 'brain profile' of a bullied child. Some children show increased vigilance and reactivity; others appear emotionally numbed or withdrawn; many show resilience, particularly when protected by supportive relationships and effective intervention.

The review also drew attention to the fact that bullying is not only about fear. It is also about belonging, social status and the ongoing effort to interpret peer behaviour. Several studies examined responses to social evaluation, inclusion or peer approval. Patterns varied, but the broader theme was that victimisation may be linked with altered responses in systems involved in reward and social evaluation. In real life, this can look like increased social monitoring, watching closely for peer cues, overthinking tone or facial expressions, or feeling highly sensitive to feedback (Ke et al., 2022).

For teachers and parents, this helps explain why some children who have been bullied may seem preoccupied with peer reactions or may react strongly to relatively small social events. These behaviours can be misunderstood as immaturity or attention-seeking, but they may reflect a nervous system working hard to navigate a social world that has previously been unpredictable and painful.

Ke and colleagues also noted findings involving prefrontal regions linked to cognitive control and regulation. In some studies, victimised young people showed patterns consistent with the increased recruitment of regulatory systems during stressful or evaluative tasks. This can be understood as increased cognitive effort: managing emotion and monitoring threat can consume mental resources that would otherwise support attention, learning and flexible thinking. In classroom terms, this can contribute to the common pattern where a child who is experiencing bullying appears distracted, forgetful or less able to cope with challenges, even if their underlying ability has not changed.

Taken together, neuroimaging research supports the broader conclusion already established in developmental stress science: repeated stress can be associated with differences in how threat, emotion and regulation systems function. However, Ke and colleagues emphasise that bullying-specific evidence is still developing. Because many studies are correlational, it is not always possible to determine whether victimisation contributes to these patterns, whether pre-existing vulnerabilities increase the risk of victimisation, or whether other stressors contribute to both. This is why the most accurate language is that peer victimisation is associated with differences in brain outcomes in some studies, rather than claiming that bullying directly causes lasting brain changes (Ke et al., 2022).

Even so, the safest conclusion remains the same: these findings point to increased vulnerability under chronic social stress, not permanent damage and not inevitable outcomes. This is also where hope sits. If the brain can adapt to threat, it can also adapt to safety. When bullying stops and children experience consistent protection, routines and supportive relationships, stress-related patterns can settle and developmental pathways can recover.

Real-life Example: Jamie's Story

Jamie (pseudonym) is nine years old. Over recent weeks, her teachers have noticed that she has become quieter in class and less engaged in her work. She appears more easily distracted, struggles to concentrate, and sometimes seems startled when spoken to unexpectedly. These changes are new and differ from how Jamie previously behaved, both socially and academically.

Further discussion reveals that Jamie has been experiencing repeated teasing from peers during break times. These incidents do not occur at set times and often take place in areas with limited adult supervision. As a result, Jamie has begun to feel unsafe during parts of the school day and remains on edge, even in the classroom.

From a developmental perspective, repeated exposure to this kind of social stress can keep a child's stress response system activated. When the body remains in a heightened state of alert, it becomes harder for the brain to prioritise learning and regulation. Systems that support attention, memory and self-control may work less effectively while stress remains high. Jamie's difficulties are therefore better understood as a response to ongoing stress, rather than a loss of ability or motivation.

Crucially, these patterns are not permanent. Research shows that when children experience safety, predictability and consistent support, stress responses can settle and cognitive functioning can improve. Jamie's story highlights both the vulnerability of the developing brain to ongoing social stress and its capacity to recover when the environment becomes more supportive.

Why This Matters

Jamie's experience reflects patterns commonly seen in educational and clinical settings. When children are exposed to repeated social threats, stress responses designed to protect them in the short term may remain active for longer than intended. This can interfere with learning, emotional regulation and social engagement, particularly during periods of active brain development.

Viewing behaviour through this lens shifts the focus away from discipline and towards understanding, protection and support. Early identification, relational safety and predictable environments play a key role in helping children regain a sense of security and restoring their capacity to learn and engage.

The next section examines how stress interacts with sleep and biological rhythms during development, and why these factors matter for both vulnerability and recovery.

What Helps Stress Systems Settle: Protective Factors and Practical Support

Understanding stress biology is only helpful if it leads to better support. The aim is not to diagnose children with a 'stressed brain', but to recognise when a child's behaviour and health may reflect prolonged social threat. The evidence reviewed in this chapter points to a simple and hopeful principle: when safety increases and stress reduces, stress-sensitive systems can begin to rebalance.

Protective factors work through several pathways. First, they reduce exposure to threat. This means stopping bullying reliably and consistently, rather than waiting for a child to 'learn resilience'. Second, they increase predictability. Predictable routines, clear boundaries and consistent adult responses reduce uncertainty, which is one of the features that makes stress feel unmanageable. Third, they increase relational safety. Supportive relationships buffer stress responses and help children regain a sense of control and belonging.

For schools, this often begins with visible adult presence in high-risk areas and times, clear reporting routes and quick follow-up. Children who are being targeted usually know which spaces are unsafe. Asking directly, calmly and without judgement can provide crucial information. It is also important to reduce the burden on the child to 'prove' what is happening. Many children minimise bullying because they fear escalation, social retaliation or being labelled as a problem.

For teachers, a stress-informed lens can change daily practice in small but meaningful ways. Children under chronic stress often struggle most during transitions, group work and unstructured tasks where social risk is higher. Support can include planned seating, careful grouping, structured choices and predictable check-ins. These adjustments are not special treatment; they are scaffolding that helps a child access learning while safeguarding work is underway.

For parents and carers, the priority is often to restore calm and predictability at home, while also working with the school to address what is happening. Children who are bullied may show irritability, shutdown, stomach aches, changes in appetite, sleep disturbance or reluctance to attend school. These can be signs of stress rather than defiance. Helpful responses include validating the child's experience ('That sounds really hard'), avoiding rapid problem-solving before the child feels heard, and keeping routines steady. Where online harassment is involved, it can help create practical boundaries around devices, particularly at night, while also ensuring the child does not feel punished for being targeted (Internet Matters, 2006).

Health professionals may see the downstream effects first: headaches, abdominal pain, sleep problems, fatigue, anxiety, low mood or school refusal. A brief, routine question about peer relationships can be clinically valuable, particularly when symptoms are recurrent or unexplained. When bullying is disclosed, the most helpful response is often a combination of validation, documentation and coordinated support with school safeguarding structures. Where a child is presenting with severe anxiety, depression, trauma symptoms or persistent physical complaints, referral pathways should be considered, but this should not replace the urgent need to stop the bullying itself.

Across all settings, it helps to keep language realistic and non-deterministic. Children do not need to hear that bullying has 'changed their brain'. They need to hear that their reactions make sense in the context of stress, that support can help, and that improvement is possible. The message is: *your body has been working hard to keep you safe, and we are going to make things safer so it does not have to work so hard.*

Finally, it is worth emphasising that recovery is often gradual. Some children settle quickly once the bullying stops; others remain watchful for a while, particularly if the bullying has been prolonged or if they have experienced multiple stressors. Consistency matters. The same protective factors that support learning, predictable routines, supportive relationships and reliable adult action are also the factors most likely to support the recalibration of stress systems over time.

Parent and Carer Support Resources

Parents and carers do not have to manage bullying alone. Specialist organisations can provide practical guidance on recognising bullying, recording incidents, communicating with schools, supporting a child emotionally and responding to online harassment. Where bullying is affecting a child's mental health, sleep, attendance or safety, parents should seek professional support.

Useful UK organisations include:

Organisation	*Support offered*	*Telephone*
Kidscape Parent Advice Line	Bullying advice for parents, carers and professionals	**0300 102 4481**
Anti-Bullying Alliance	Anti-bullying guidance and signposting	**020 7843 6000, voice message service**

Organisation	*Support offered*	*Telephone*
NSPCC Helpline	For adults worried about a child	**0808 800 5000**
Childline	Confidential support for children and young people	**0800 1111**
YoungMinds Parents Helpline	Parent support for young people's mental health	**0808 802 5544**
PAPYRUS HOPELINE247	Support for young people experiencing suicidal thoughts, or anyone worried about a young person	**0300 102 2470, text HOPE to 88247**
Samaritans	24-hour emotional support	**116 123**
Emergency services	Immediate risk of harm	**999**
NHS urgent advice	Urgent health or mental health advice when it is not a 999 emergency	**111**
Find a Helpline	International directory of verified helplines for mental health, suicide prevention, bullying, abuse, self-harm, trauma, stress and related concerns	Visit **findahelpline.com** and select your country

Note: Contact details can change. Readers should check each organisation's website for current opening hours and access options. If a child is at immediate risk of harm, call 999 in the UK, attend the nearest emergency department, or contact the relevant emergency service in your country. For readers outside the UK, Find a Helpline provides an international directory of verified support services by country and topic.
Sources: Anti-Bullying Alliance (2026), Childline (2026), Find a Helpline (2026), Kidscape (2026), NSPCC (2026), PAPYRUS (2026) and YoungMinds (2026).

Key Takeaways

- Not all stress is harmful; problems arise when threat is repeated, unpredictable or inescapable.
- Bullying can keep the body in 'on alert' mode, which affects learning and regulation
- Stress changes are often adaptive in the moment, but unhelpful when they don't switch off
- Sleep and safety are not 'nice to have'; they're core to recovery
- Brain findings should guide support, not become a story of permanent damage

References

Anti-Bullying Alliance (2026) *Advice for parents and carers*. Available at: https://anti-bullyingalliance.org.uk/ (Accessed: 26 May 2026).

Arain, M., Haque, M., Johal, L., Mathur, P., Nel, W., Rais, A. and Sharma, S. (2013) 'Maturation of the adolescent brain', *Neuropsychiatric Disease and Treatment*, 9, pp. 449–461.

Arnsten, A.F.T. (2015) 'Stress weakens prefrontal networks: Molecular insults to higher cognition', *Nature Reviews Neuroscience*, 16(10), pp. 605–621.

Arnsten, A.F.T., Joyce, M.K.P. and Roberts, A.C. (2023) 'The aversive lens: Stress effects on the prefrontal–cingulate cortical pathways that regulate emotion', *Neuroscience and Biobehavioral Reviews*, 149, 105148.

Arseneault, L. (2018) 'Annual research review: The persistent and pervasive impact of being bullied in childhood and adolescence: Implications for policy and practice', *Journal of Child Psychology and Psychiatry*, 59(4), pp. 405–421.

Bethlehem, R.A.I., Seidlitz, J., White, S.R., Vogel, J.W., Anderson, K.M., Adamson, C., Adler, S., Alexopoulos, G.S., Anagnostou, E., Areces-Gonzalez, A., Astle, D.E., Auyeung, B., Ayub, M., Bae, J., Ball, G., Baron-Cohen, S., Beare, R., Bedford, S.A., Benegal, V., Beyer, F., Blangero, J., Blesa Cábez, M., Boardman, J.P., Borzage, M., Bosch-Bayard, J.F., Bourke, N., Calhoun, V.D., Chakravarty, M.M., Chen, C., Chertavian, C., Chételat, G., Chong, Y.S., Cole, J.H., Corvin, A., Costantino, M., Courchesne, E., Crivello, F., Cropley, V.L., Crosbie, J., Crossley, N., Delarue, M., Delorme, R., Desrivières, S., Devenyi, G.A., Di Biase, M.A., Dolan, R., Donald, K.A., Donohoe, G., Dunlop, K., Edwards, A.D., Elison, J.T., Ellis, C.T., Elman, J.A., Eyler, L., Fair, D.A., Feczko, E., Fletcher, P.C., Fonagy, P., Franz, C.E., Galan-Garcia, L., Gholipour, A., Giedd, J., Gilmore, J.H., Glahn, D.C., Goodyer, I.M., Grant, P.E., Groenewold, N.A., Gunning, F.M., Gur, R.E., Gur, R.C., Hammill, C.F., Hansson, O., Hedden, T., Heinz, A., Henson, R.N., Heuer, K., Hoare, J., Holla, B., Holmes, A.J., Holt, R., Huang, H., Im, K., Ipser, J., Jack, C.R. Jr, Jackowski, A.P., Jia, T., Johnson, K.A., Jones, P.B., Jones, D.T., Kahn, R.S., Karlsson, H., Karlsson, L., Kawashima, R., Kelley, E.A., Kern, S., Kim, K.W., Kitzbichler, M.G., Kremen, W.S., Lalonde, F., Landeau, B., Lee, S., Lerch, J., Lewis, J.D., Li, J., Liao, W., Liston, C., Lombardo, M.V., Lv, J., Lynch, C., Mallard, T.T., Marcelis, M., Markello, R.D., Mathias, S.R., Mazoyer, B., McGuire, P., Meaney, M.J., Mechelli, A., Medic, N., Misic, B., Morgan, S.E., Mothersill, D., Nigg, J., Ong, M.Q.W., Ortinau, C., Ossenkoppele, R., Ouyang, M., Palaniyappan, L., Paly, L., Pan, P.M., Pantelis, C., Park, M.M., Paus, T., Pausova, Z., Paz-Linares, D., Pichet Binette, A., Pierce, K., Qian, X., Qiu, J., Qiu, A., Raznahan, A., Rittman, T., Rodrigue, A., Rollins, C.K., Romero-Garcia, R., Ronan, L., Rosenberg, M.D., Rowitch, D.H., Salum, G.A., Satterthwaite, T.D., Schaare, H.L., Schachar, R.J., Schultz, A.P., Schumann, G., Schöll, M., Sharp, D., Shinohara, R.T., Skoog, I., Smyser, C.D., Sperling, R.A., Stein, D.J., Stolicyn, A., Suckling, J., Sullivan, G., Taki, Y., Thyreau, B., Toro, R., Traut, N., Tsvetanov, K.A., Turk-Browne, N.B., Tuulari, J.J., Tzourio, C., Vachon-Presseau, É., Valdes-Sosa, M.J., Valdes-Sosa, P.A., Valk, S.L., van Amelsvoort, T., Vandekar, S.N., Vasung, L., Victoria, L.W., Villeneuve, S., Villringer, A., Vértes, P.E., Wagstyl, K., Wang, Y.S., Warfield, S.K., Warrier, V., Westman, E., Westwater, M.L., Whalley, H.C., Witte, A.V., Yang, N., Yeo, B., Yun, H., Zalesky, A., Zar, H.J., Zettergren, A., Zhou, J.H., Ziauddeen, H., Zugman, A. and

Zuo, X.N. (2022) 'Brain charts for the human lifespan', *Nature*, 604(7906), pp. 525–533.

Childline (2026) *Bullying and cyberbullying*. Available at: www.childline.org.uk/ (Accessed: 26 May 2026).

Find a Helpline (2026) *Suicide hotlines and crisis helplines: Free, 24/7 chat, text and phone support*. Available at: https://findahelpline.com/ (Accessed: 26 May 2026).

Gee, D.G., Cohodes, E.M., McLaughlin, K.A. and Telzer, E.H. (2021) 'Leveraging developmental neuroscience to understand the impact of adversity on youth', *Developmental Cognitive Neuroscience*, 47, 100889.

Girotti, M., Bulin, S.E. and Carreno, F.R. (2024) 'Effects of chronic stress on cognitive function – from neurobiology to intervention', *Neurobiology of Stress*, 33, 100670.

Gregory, A.M., Kivelä, L., Barclay, N.L., Reynolds, S. and Forbes, E.E. (2024) 'Sleep, stress and emotional regulation during adolescence', *Neuroscience and Biobehavioral Reviews*, 156, 105453.

Internet Matters (2026) *Cyberbullying advice hub*. Available at: www.internetmatters.org/ (Accessed: 26 May 2026).

Ke, T., De Simoni, S., Barker, E.D. and Smith, P. (2022) 'The association between peer-victimisation and structural and functional brain outcomes: A systematic review', *JCPP Advances*, 2, e12081. doi:10.1002/jcv2.12081.

Kidscape (2026) *Help with bullying*. Available at: www.kidscape.org.uk/ (Accessed: 26 May 2026).

Lupien, S.J., Juster, R.-P. and McEwen, B.S. (2018) 'The effects of chronic stress on the human brain: From neurotoxicity, to vulnerability, to opportunity', *Neuroscience and Biobehavioral Reviews*, 85, pp. 1–15.

McEwen, B.S. (2017) 'Neurobiological and systemic effects of chronic stress', *Chronic Stress*, 1, pp. 1–11. doi:10.1177/2470547017692328.

McLaughlin, K.A., Weissman, D. and Bitrán, D. (2019) 'Childhood adversity and neural development: A systematic review', *Annual Review of Developmental Psychology*, 1, pp. 277–312. doi:10.1146/annurev-devpsych-121318-084950.

Menken, M.S., Rodriguez Rivera, P.J., Isaiah, A., Ernst, T., Cloak, C.C. and Chang, L. (2023) 'Longitudinal alterations in brain morphometry mediated the effects of bullying victimization on cognitive development in preadolescents', *Developmental Cognitive Neuroscience*, 61, 101247. doi:10.1016/j.dcn.2023.101247.

Miller, G.E., Chen, E. and Parker, K.J. (2011) 'Psychological stress in childhood and susceptibility to the chronic diseases of aging: Moving toward a model of behavioral and biological mechanisms', *Psychological Bulletin*, 137(6), pp. 959–997. doi:10.1037/a0024768.

Moseley, R.L., Camacho, M.C., Gregory, A.M., Fairchild, G. and Barker, E.D. (2022) 'Stress exposure and inefficiency of executive control networks in adolescence', *NeuroImage*, 252, 119041.

Moseley, R.L., Gregory, A.M., Fairchild, G. and Barker, E.D. (2024) 'Developmental stress and large-scale brain network reorganisation', *Biological Psychiatry*, 95(3), pp. 245–256.

NSPCC (2026) *Bullying and cyberbullying*. Available at: www.nspcc.org.uk/ (Accessed: 26 May 2026).

OpenStax College (2013) *Anatomy & physiology*. Rice University. (Image source used in Figure 2.1 via Wikimedia Commons, CC BY 3.0).
Orben, A., Meier, A., Dalgleish, T. and Blakemore, S.-J. (2024) 'Mechanisms linking social media use to adolescent mental health vulnerability', Nature Mental Health. doi:10.1038/s44159-024-00307-y.
PAPYRUS (2026) *HOPELINE247*. Available at: www.papyrus-uk.org/ (Accessed: 26 May 2026).
Servier Medical Art (n.d.) *Brain: hippocampus*. Available at: https://smart.servier.com/smart_image/hippocampus/ (Accessed: 30 July 2026).
Shonkoff, J.P., Garner, A.S. and the Committee on Psychosocial Aspects of Child and Family Health, Committee on Early Childhood, Adoption, and Dependent Care and Section on Developmental and Behavioral Pediatrics (2012) 'The lifelong effects of early childhood adversity and toxic stress', *Pediatrics*, 129(1), pp. e232–e246. doi: 10.1542/peds.2011-2663.
Shonkoff, J.P., Slopen, N. and Williams, D.R. (2021) 'Early childhood adversity, toxic stress, and the impacts of racism on the foundations of health', *Annual Review of Public Health*, 42, pp. 115–134. doi:10.1146/annurev-publhealth-090419-101940.
Short, M.A., Booth, S.A., Omar, O., Ostlundh, L. and Arora, T. (2023) 'Sleep duration and mental health in adolescents: Cross-sectional and longitudinal evidence', *Journal of Adolescent Health*, 72(2), pp. 215–223.
Suglia, S.F., Appleton, A.A., Bleil, M.E., Campo, R.A., Dube, S.R., Fagundes, C.P., Heard-Garris, N.J., Johnson, S.B., Slopen, N., Stoney, C.M. and Watamura, S.E. (2021) 'Timing, duration, and differential susceptibility to early life adversities and cardiovascular disease risk across the lifespan: Implications for future research', *Preventive Medicine*, 153, 106736. doi:10.1016/j.ypmed.2021.106736.
Takizawa, R., Maughan, B. and Arseneault, L. (2014) 'Adult health outcomes of childhood bullying victimization: Evidence from a five-decade longitudinal British birth cohort', *American Journal of Psychiatry*, 171(7), pp. 777–784. doi:10.1176/appi.ajp.2014.13101401.
Tamnes, C.K., Herting, M.M., Goddings, A.L., Meuwese, R., Blakemore, S.J., Dahl, R.E., Güroğlu, B., Raznahan, A., Sowell, E.R., Crone, E.A. and Mills, K.L. (2017) 'Development of the cerebral cortex across adolescence: A multisample study of inter-related longitudinal changes in cortical volume, surface area, and thickness', *The Journal of Neuroscience*, 37(12), pp. 3402–3412. doi:10.1523/JNEUROSCI.3302-16.2017.
Teicher, M.H., Samson, J.A., Anderson, C.M. and Ohashi, K. (2016) 'The effects of childhood maltreatment on brain structure, function and connectivity', *Nature Reviews Neuroscience*, 17(10), pp. 652–666. doi:10.1038/nrn.2016.111.
Vaillancourt, T., Hymel, S. and McDougall, P. (2013) 'The biological underpinnings of peer victimization: Understanding why and how the effects of bullying can last a lifetime', *Theory Into Practice*, 52(4), pp. 241–248. doi:10.1080/00405841.2013.829726.
Washington Irving (2020) *Hippocampus.svg*. Wikimedia Commons. Available at: https://commons.wikimedia.org/wiki/File:Hippocampus.svg (Accessed: 26 May 2026).

Wolke, D., Copeland, W.E., Angold, A. and Costello, E.J. (2013) 'Impact of bullying in childhood on adult health, wealth, crime, and social outcomes', *Psychological Science*, 24(10), pp. 1958–1970. doi:10.1177/0956797613481608.
Wolke, D. and Lereya, S.T. (2015) 'Long-term effects of bullying', *Archives of Disease in Childhood*, 100(9), pp. 879–885.
YoungMinds (2026) *Bullying*. Available at: www.youngminds.org.uk/ (Accessed: 26 May 2026).

Chapter 3

How Bullying Affects the Brain

Abstract

This chapter explains how bullying can affect the developing brain, not as a simple story of damage, but as a stress-based developmental process that varies widely between children. Repeated peer victimisation can function as sustained social threat, engaging systems involved in danger detection, emotional regulation, learning and social belonging. For some children, especially when bullying is chronic, humiliating and difficult to escape, stress responses may remain activated, reducing opportunities for recovery and contributing to difficulties with sleep, attention, memory and mood. The chapter emphasises nuance and causality: some children have pre-existing traits that increase the likelihood of being targeted. Bullying can then intensify these vulnerabilities over time. It also outlines the distinct needs of children who are both bullied and bully others, whose profiles often involve heightened dysregulation and complex peer positioning. Throughout, the focus remains on probability rather than certainty, and on the potential for recovery when safety, support and predictable environments are restored.

In This Chapter

- Bullying as a sustained social threat, why the brain treats exclusion as serious
- Why some children look 'fine' outwardly, but carry high stress internally
- Common patterns (sleep, attention, mood, learning, confidence) and why they vary
- Bidirectional pathways: what can increase risk, and what bullying can intensify
- What helps most when a child is stuck in ongoing stress

DOI: 10.4324/9781003771777-5

A Note on Language

Throughout this book, person-first language is used wherever possible: children who are bullied, children who bully, and children who are both bullied and bully others. Research literature often uses terms such as victim, perpetrator or bully-victim. While analytically useful, such labels can become fixed identities. A child described solely as a victim may begin to see themselves as powerless; a child repeatedly described as a bully may internalise that description. Language shapes expectation. By emphasising behaviour and experience rather than identity, the focus remains on development, accountability and change.

Building on the neurodevelopmental processes outlined in Chapter 2, this chapter examines how repeated peer victimisation may influence brain-linked functioning across childhood and adolescence. The aim is not to suggest that bullying inevitably 'changes the brain' in a permanent or uniform way. Rather, repeated victimisation can increase strain on systems that support threat detection, emotional regulation, learning and social belonging (McLaughlin et al., 2014). When bullying is persistent, especially when it is humiliating, unpredictable and difficult to escape, stress-related adaptations may become more persistent and begin to interfere with attention, memory, sleep and social confidence.

A balanced account also requires careful attention to causality. Much of the evidence in this field is correlational, and bullying commonly co-occurs with other sources of stress and vulnerability (Arseneault et al., 2010). Some differences observed in studies may also precede victimisation, reflecting traits that increase the likelihood of being targeted. This chapter therefore uses cautious, evidence-aligned language, emphasising probability rather than certainty (Arseneault, 2018). It also highlights recovery: many children improve substantially when safety is restored, supportive relationships are strengthened and stress is reduced.

Bullying as a Sustained Social Threat

Why the Brain Takes Peer Threat Seriously

Bullying is a developmental stressor with a particular social signature. For children and adolescents, peer belonging is closely tied to safety, identity and everyday functioning. Repeated exclusion, public humiliation, intimidation and online harassment can signal that a child's position within the peer group is unsafe. When those signals are repeated, the child may begin to anticipate danger in environments that previously felt neutral, corridors, lunchtime spaces, group work, the bus or online group chats.

This helps explain why adults sometimes underestimate the impact of incidents that appear, in isolation, to be 'minor'. The stress response is shaped not only by the content of an incident, but by repetition, power imbalance and whether the child experiences realistic routes to protection. Bullying is often less of an isolated event than an ongoing social position that can narrow a child's sense of safety and control.

The Role of Predictability, Humiliation and Audience

The features that most reliably increase stress load are those that reduce predictability and increase exposure: bullying that is unpredictable, public, humiliating and difficult to escape. An 'audience' can amplify distress because it increases shame and the fear of reputational damage. This is one reason cyberbullying can be experienced as particularly intense: the audience may be large or unknown, and content can be shared or revisited. When a child believes that peers have defined them in a negative way, they may monitor social cues constantly in an attempt to prevent further injury.

Stress Thresholds: Acute Distress, Chronic Strain and Trauma-like Responses

Acute Distress and Early Warning Signs

In the early stages, children who experience bullying often show changes in mood, behaviour and social engagement. These responses are not signs of weakness or pathology, but adaptive attempts to cope with perceived threat. Common early reactions include increased anxiety, withdrawal from peers, irritability, heightened emotional sensitivity and reduced participation in classroom activities. Physical complaints such as headaches, stomach aches or fatigue are frequently reported, particularly among younger children who may struggle to express emotional distress verbally.

Adults may observe declining concentration, avoidance of specific spaces or routines or reluctance to attend school. These reactions are often context-dependent: some children appear relatively settled at home but are dysregulated on school mornings; others maintain composure at school, but 'release' distress in the evening. Importantly, when bullying is addressed promptly, and safety is restored, many children improve significantly, underscoring the value of early identification and intervention.

Chronic Strain and Trauma-like Responses

While many children experience transient distress, a smaller proportion develop more severe and persistent responses. Risk increases when bullying is chronic, unpredictable, socially humiliating or experienced as inescapable, especially when children feel unsupported or unheard. For some children, repeated bullying may be experienced as traumatic. Symptoms can include intrusive thoughts or memories, sleep disruption, heightened anxiety, emotional numbing, exaggerated fear responses and persistent shame or helplessness. These reactions may resemble trauma-related patterns, although not all affected children meet the diagnostic criteria for post-traumatic stress disorder.

Emerging longitudinal evidence supports the observation that, for a subset of young people, trauma-related symptom clusters may become a key driver of later mood and anxiety difficulties. Cross-lagged analyses in adolescents and emerging adults with bullying victimisation histories indicate that complex post-traumatic stress disorder (CPTSD) symptoms can more strongly predict later depression and anxiety than the reverse direction, while still allowing for reciprocal effects (Liu et al., 2025). This is best understood as a risk pathway rather than an inevitability: persistent hypervigilance, negative self-concept and dysregulation can consolidate and sustain vulnerability over time.

Typical Distress versus Trauma Responses: Avoiding Over- or Under-Pathologising

It is possible to recognise that bullying can be traumatic for some children without assuming that all bullying leads to trauma. Equally, it is possible to acknowledge that a child does not meet a diagnostic threshold while still recognising that their functioning has been significantly affected. A trauma-informed stance is less about applying labels and more about asking practical questions: How often is the child's sense of safety being threatened? Do they have reliable routes back to calm? Are adults consistently interrupting harm and restoring dignity?

Stress Response Systems and Brain-linked Functioning

From Threat to Functioning: What Changes from Day To Day

The brain does not respond to bullying 'directly'; it responds to bullying as social danger (McLaughlin et al., 2021). When a child anticipates threat, stress pathways activate to support rapid responding and learning about what to avoid. In the short term, this can be adaptive. The difficulty arises when activation becomes frequent and prolonged, especially if the child has limited access to protection and recovery (Shonkoff et al., 2012; McEwen, 2017).

To avoid repeating the detailed physiology covered in Chapter 2, the focus here is on functional consequences. When threat systems dominate, children may show narrowed attention, increased reactivity, reduced working memory and difficulty shifting out of defensive states. This can present as 'not listening', 'overreacting', 'being oppositional' or 'switching off'. The more accurate interpretation is often that the child's system is prioritising safety over flexibility.

Cortisol Findings: Why Results Vary and What that Means in Practice

Research findings on stress biology in bullied children vary (Vaillancourt et al., 2013). Some studies report heightened cortisol responses to psychosocial stress, while others suggest altered or blunted patterns under conditions of chronic exposure. Both heightened and blunted patterns may indicate dysregulation, depending on context, timing and individual sensitivity (Chen et al., 2018; Du Plessis et al., 2019). For practice, the key point is not the direction of cortisol change, but the functional picture: disrupted sleep, persistent vigilance, emotional volatility and reduced recovery time.

Brain Networks Relevant to Bullying-related Stress

Threat Detection and Salience

Systems involved in detecting potential danger and assigning emotional significance to cues may become more sensitive when a child has been repeatedly targeted (Gong et al., 2024). Social cues can become loaded: laughter nearby, a whisper, a message notification or a group forming. This can present as vigilance, irritability, rapid escalation or avoidance. Systematic review evidence suggests that peer-victimisation is associated with structural and functional brain differences in some studies, although findings are mixed and confounded by multiple factors (Ke et al., 2022).

Social Pain and Rejection Sensitivity

Exclusion and humiliation can activate networks involved in social distress and self-evaluation. Repeated experiences of rejection may increase rejection sensitivity, leading children to anticipate negative evaluation and withdraw, mask, or appease, even in safer contexts. This is particularly relevant for relational bullying, where the injury is often to belonging and reputation rather than physical safety.

Emotion Regulation and Control

Prefrontal systems support inhibition, perspective-taking and the regulation of emotional reactions. Under sustained stress, children may struggle to access these capacities in real time. This is not a matter of willpower; it reflects the difficulty of maintaining regulation under threat, particularly while regulatory systems are still developing. For practice, the implication is that co-regulation (adult calm, predictability and supportive limit-setting) is often more effective than escalation and punishment for stress-driven behaviour.

How Heightened Threat Sensitivity Can Look in Everyday Life

For parents and teachers, the relevance of these networks is functional rather than anatomical. When a child's brain is repeatedly asked to evaluate social safety, they may begin to respond as though danger is likely, even when it is uncertain. Some children become hypervigilant, scanning faces, monitoring tone and tracking group movement. In class, they may track who is looking at them rather than what the teacher is saying and may overinterpret ambiguous cues as threatening. Other children show shutdown or withdrawal. When threat feels chronic and inescapable, reducing engagement can become a form of protection. This can appear as 'going quiet', disengaging from group work or avoiding participation.

Why these Patterns are Often Misunderstood

Adults may interpret hypervigilance as attitude ('always looking for trouble') or interpret shutdown as laziness ('not trying'). Both interpretations can increase shame and reduce disclosure. A more helpful stance is curiosity: What does the behaviour protect the child from? When is it most likely to occur? Which contexts feel safest? This approach supports practical, protective intervention rather than escalation.

Learning, Attention and Memory: When School becomes Harder

Safety versus Learning Priorities

When school is a setting of threat, the brain prioritises safety over learning (Wade et al., 2022). This can look like reduced working memory during lessons, difficulty concentrating in unstructured times, shutdown or 'zoning out', and increasing avoidance of school. These patterns are often misinterpreted as poor motivation or behaviour. A stress-informed interpretation is more accurate: cognitive resources are being diverted towards monitoring risk.

Why Bullying can be Misread as 'Attention Problems'

Bullying-related stress can mimic or amplify difficulties that look like attention problems, learning difficulties or oppositional behaviour. A child who appears distracted may be allocating attention to threat-monitoring. A child who repeatedly asks to leave the classroom may be trying to avoid unstructured peer contact. A child who becomes irritable at specific times of the day may be anticipating a bullying hotspot such as lining up, lunch, change rooms or the journey home.

A helpful adult question is: 'What is this behaviour doing for the child?' In many cases, it is helping them avoid humiliation, regain a sense of control or reduce fear. This reframing supports responses that prioritise safety planning, predictable routines, adult supervision at hotspots and supportive relationships, alongside any needed learning support.

The Cost of Misinterpretation

When adults respond only to surface behaviour, punishing, removing privileges or labelling the child as 'difficult' can increase the stress load, and regulation of stress can worsen. This can create a cascade: more distress leads to more dysregulation, which leads to more sanctions, which reduces belonging and increases vulnerability. Recognising bullying-related stress early can prevent these secondary harms.

School Engagement and Longer-term Educational Trajectories

Bullying-related stress can affect educational engagement through multiple pathways. In the short term, fear and vigilance reduce concentration and participation. Over time, some children begin to avoid school entirely, particularly when bullying occurs in unstructured settings or when disclosures do not lead to effective action. School avoidance is rarely a 'choice' in the ordinary sense; it is often the outcome of repeated experiences of threat without adequate protection.

When disengagement continues, academic attainment can be affected through missed instruction, reduced confidence and fewer opportunities for mastery. These patterns can be misread as lack of motivation, rather than be recognised as indicators of distress. A supportive school response therefore needs to address both safety and learning access: re-establishing protected routines, adjusting timetables temporarily, supporting re-entry and ensuring that the child can engage without being repeatedly exposed to harm.

Social Cue Processing and Heightened Monitoring

Cohort Findings and Cautious Interpretation

Large cohort studies suggest that frequent bullying involvement is associated with differences in brain morphology in some regions that are linked to social cue processing. One example is a thicker cortex in the fusiform gyrus among children frequently involved in bullying as targets, compared to uninvolved peers (Muetzel et al., 2019). Such findings do not establish causation. However, they support a plausible interpretation: repeated exposure to social threat can increase attention to faces and expressions, making some children more attuned to subtle cues of ridicule or exclusion.

Social Monitoring as a Learned Skill with a Cost

Some bullied children become exceptionally skilled at reading micro-signals: who is looking, who is laughing, who is forming a group? This can reduce surprise and help them avoid hotspots. The cost is cognitive and emotional: constant monitoring reduces attention available for learning and can sustain fatigue, irritability and avoidance. Adults can help by reducing hotspots and providing predictable, supportive supervision that lowers the child's need to self-protect in this way.

Brain Morphology and Cognition: What Cohort Studies Suggest

Longitudinal Findings

Longitudinal cohort research has begun to examine bullying involvement alongside brain morphometry and cognition. Findings suggest associations between prolonged victimisation and differences in regional volume, surface area and cortical thickness, alongside poorer cognitive performance in some samples (Menken et al., 2023). The direction of effects is not uniform across regions, and results vary by measurement and developmental stage. These nuances matter: the presence of 'differences' does not reveal whether a change is harmful, compensatory or shaped by earlier vulnerability.

Why Developmental Timing Matters

Bullying does not occur in a developmental vacuum. The same experience can have different implications depending on age, the developmental tasks of that stage, and available support (Sayler et al., 2025). In middle childhood, peer acceptance becomes increasingly important, yet children still rely heavily on adults to interpret social meaning and restore safety. Victimisation during this stage can interfere with growing competence, classroom confidence and willingness to take learning risks. In adolescence, peer evaluation becomes more salient, and identity development accelerates. Bullying may be experienced as an attack on identity and social status, especially when it occurs publicly or online. Adolescents may also conceal what is happening due to fears about reputation or retaliation.

Plasticity and Recovery: What Changes when Safety Returns

A key message for this chapter is that stress-related adaptations are not fixed. When children experience reliable protection, supportive relationships and reduced exposure to threat, many stress-linked patterns begin to settle. Practically, this may look like improved sleep, fewer physical complaints, reduced vigilance, and a return of curiosity and engagement. Recovery is often uneven: some children appear to improve quickly once bullying stops, while others continue to show fear and avoidance for longer, particularly if the bullying was prolonged or if it intersected with earlier adversity. Adults can support recovery by anticipating that the child may remain 'on edge', even after the bullying has been addressed, and by maintaining predictable protection long enough for safety learning to consolidate.

Different Forms of Bullying and Coping Under Threat

Physical, Relational and Cyberbullying: Different Loads

Bullying is not a single exposure. Different forms of bullying can place different cognitive and emotional demands on children (Wen et al., 2023). Physical bullying can create direct fear and anticipatory stress, increasing scanning of the environment and avoidance of routes and spaces. Relational bullying, exclusion, rumour, humiliation and social sabotage targets belonging and identity. Because it is often ambiguous and socially complex, it can lead to prolonged rumination: 'Who is safe? What did I do? Who is saying what?' Cyberbullying can combine intensity with inescapability. Even when messages stop, the child may continue to check their devices to regain certainty, which reduces recovery time and disrupts sleep.

Executive Functioning, Anxiety and Problematic Internet Use

Online peer stress can become difficult to regulate when adolescents are already managing elevated anxiety or weaker executive-function skills. Executive functions include inhibitory control, working memory and cognitive flexibility. These skills support judgement, pause-and-think capacity and emotion regulation, especially under social pressure. When a young person is under threat, executive systems may be less available, and coping can shift toward short-term relief rather than long-term wellbeing.

Evidence from a representative adolescent sample indicates that problematic internet use is associated with anxiety, cyberbullying involvement and executive-function difficulties (Real-Fernández et al., 2025). This does not mean that executive-function differences 'cause' bullying or that problematic use is inevitable for bullied adolescents. Instead, the findings fit a contextual model: when a young person feels unsafe in face-to-face peer settings, online spaces may provide a substitute for belonging or distraction. At the same time, greater online exposure can amplify vulnerability to further harassment, rumination and monitoring behaviours, reducing recovery time and compounding sleep disruption.

Reducing Digital Harm while Protecting Belonging

Digital safeguarding is most effective when paired with belonging and support. Simply removing devices may reduce exposure in the short term, but can also increase social isolation if peers organise socially online. A more protective approach is collaborative: helping young people identify safe peers and spaces, creating plans for reporting and blocking, and reducing nighttime access to triggering content. Where cyberbullying intersects with school peer groups, coordinated school responses are often necessary to prevent harm from being treated as 'outside school' and therefore unaddressed.

Risk-taking and 'Fast Relief' Coping

Some adolescents cope with bullying-related shame or fear by moving toward behaviours that provide fast relief or rapid status repair. This can include risk-taking, impulsive retaliation online, substance use or aligning with peers who offer protection but increase exposure to conflict. Adults can reduce risk by addressing the function of the behaviour, offering protection, certainty or belonging, while strengthening safer routes to those needs.

Self-esteem and Self-concept as Mechanisms

Self-esteem as a Pathway to Anxiety and Depression

Alongside stress responses and threat processing, bullying can shape development through its effects on self-esteem and self-concept. Self-esteem is not simply 'confidence'; it is a child's sense of worth, social value, competence and belonging. When bullying is repeated, particularly when it is humiliating or identity-focused, children may internalise negative messages: 'I am unlikeable', 'I am powerless', 'something is wrong with me'. Over time, these beliefs can shape the interpretation of future interactions and willingness to seek support.

Modelling studies indicate that self-esteem can function as a key pathway that links bullying victimisation to anxiety and depression. In a structural equation model, self-esteem mediated the association between victimisation and both anxiety and depressive symptoms, with the mediated pathway being particularly important for depression (Balluerka et al., 2023). This supports a non-deterministic explanation: bullying does not cause depression or anxiety in isolation, but can increase risk by undermining the psychological and relational scaffolding that supports regulation and belonging.

High-risk and Avoidant Coping, including Digital Escape

Some young people cope with bullying-related distress through behaviours that offer rapid relief, but increase longer-term risk, such as substance use, school avoidance or impulsive risk-taking. Less visible coping can include excessive digital engagement, particularly when online spaces become a substitute for safety, distraction or connection. Longitudinal research indicates that bullying victimisation can contribute to later mobile phone addiction through emotional distress, with depression and social anxiety acting as mediators and with gender differences in the relative strength of these pathways (Li et al., 2025). A non-moralising interpretation is important: problematic digital use can reflect attempts to manage threat and isolation, and support may need to target underlying anxiety, low mood, sleep disruption and online safety together.

Bullying, Low self-esteem and Psychotic-like Experiences: A Cautious Note For Clinicians

Most children who are bullied will not develop severe psychiatric outcomes. However, for health professionals, it is useful to acknowledge that peer victimisation can be associated with broader mental health vulnerability in some contexts, particularly when it is prolonged, combined with other adversity, and experienced alongside low self-esteem and social defeat (Evans-Lacko et al., 2017). A study examining bullying exposure and self-esteem in relation to psychotic-like experiences and clinical high-risk status reported higher bullying exposure and lower self-esteem among groups at elevated psychosis risk, compared with a non-risk group (Domínguez et al., 2025).

This should be framed carefully. The most defensible interpretation is that bullying exposure may function as a stress-related risk marker for a small subset of young people, and that associations may be bidirectional: young people who already experience unusual perceptual experiences, heightened anxiety or social vulnerability may also be more likely to be targeted. The clinical implication is therefore not that bullying 'causes psychosis', but that bullying exposure should be included in the formulation when a young person presents with significant distress, paranoia-like fears, unusual experiences or functional decline. The practical response remains protective and relational: reduce exposure, restore safety, and address shame and isolation.

Social Trust, Attachment and Longer-term Relational Patterns

A child's sense of social safety is built through repeated experiences of protection and belonging. When bullying is prolonged and unbuffered, it may shape expectations about whether others are safe, whether disclosure is worthwhile, and whether relationships are reliable. Some young people respond by withdrawing; others respond by becoming highly vigilant in relationships, expecting rejection. Longer-term studies suggest that bullying histories can be associated with later difficulties in trust and social connection, although outcomes remain variable and are influenced by later protective relationships (Takizawa et al., 2014; Wolke and Lereya, 2015). For practice, this reinforces the value of ensuring that bullied children experience at least one relationship in which they are believed and protected, because that experience can counteract the expectation that 'people will not help'.

Risk, Vulnerability and Bidirectional Causality

Pre-existing Traits and Transactional Pathways

Understanding bullying-related outcomes requires explicit attention to bidirectional processes. Some children have pre-existing characteristics, such as heightened anxiety sensitivity, behavioural inhibition, neurodevelopmental differences or executive-function challenges, that can increase their likelihood of being targeted by peers, particularly in environments where difference is exploited and adult protection is inconsistent. Bullying can then exacerbate those vulnerabilities, creating a feedback loop in which distress increases exposure to further victimisation (Schoeler et al., 2019).

Genetic Susceptibility and Peer Dynamics

Bidirectional pathways are consistent with evidence that some individual differences may precede bullying involvement. A longitudinal study using peer nominations in early childhood found that a polygenic risk score derived from a conduct disorder genome-wide association study was associated with membership in bullying involvement profiles (Musci et al., 2018). This does not imply that genetics determines bullying behaviour or victimisation, nor does it reduce accountability. Rather, it supports an interactional model in which pre-existing differences in regulation and social functioning can shape peer dynamics and exposure to risk, while victimisation can intensify dysregulation and distress.

A Practical Formulation Framework for Professionals

For health professionals, educators and pastoral teams, a formulation approach helps translate the bidirectional model into targeted action without blame. A practical structure is: (1) exposure profile (what is happening, how often, where, and with what audience); (2) vulnerability and context (factors that increase the likelihood of targeting or intensify impact); (3) protective factors (trusted adults, friendships, structured belonging); (4) current stress load (sleep, appetite, concentration, mood, attendance); (5) coping pattern (withdrawal, masking, retaliation, risk-taking, digital escape); (6) function of behaviour (avoid humiliation, regain control, reduce fear); and (7) intervention targets (immediate environmental protection plus support for regulation and recovery).

This structure supports interprofessional coordination. Schools can focus on safety planning, hotspot supervision, reporting pathways and peer-group dynamics. Health services can address anxiety, mood, trauma-like symptoms, sleep disruption and risk indicators, while helping families navigate systems. The child's experience should remain central, and adults should take responsibility for changing environments rather than placing the burden on the child to 'cope better' in an unsafe context.

Children Who are Both Bullied and Bully Others

A Distinct and Higher-need Profile

Children who are both bullied and bully others (often termed bully-victims in the research literature) frequently show a different behavioural and emotional profile from children who are only bullied or only bully (Wolke et al., 2013). They are more likely to experience emotional dysregulation, peer rejection and co-occurring difficulties, and may cycle between vulnerability and reactive aggression. Their behaviour can reflect a complex mixture of threat reactivity, status-seeking, learned aggression and attempts to regain control in unsafe environments.

Implications for Intervention and Risk Management

This does not remove accountability for harm, but suggests that purely punitive responses are unlikely to be effective. Intervention typically needs to combine clear boundaries and repair (addressing harm caused) with relational and regulation-focused support (addressing stress load, skills gaps and exposure to victimisation). Clinically, it is important to assess for co-occurring anxiety, trauma-like symptoms, neurodevelopmental needs and any safety risks, while schools often need to adjust supervision and peer-group structures.

Where bullying involvement is complex, adults may also need to address group processes. Some peer groups reward dominance and humiliation. In these contexts, individual behaviour plans are not sufficient without changes to peer norms, supervision and school-wide messaging about dignity and safety. A consistent, adult-led response increases predictability and reduces the reward of bullying within the peer hierarchy.

Puberty, Appearance-related Victimisation and Developmental Vulnerability

Pubertal Asynchrony as a Contextual Risk Factor

Pubertal change can alter peer dynamics by increasing attention to appearance and social comparison. Recent research highlights pubertal asynchrony (variation in the timing of different pubertal milestones) as a potential vulnerability context for appearance-related victimisation. In a study of adolescents aged 10–16, greater pubertal asynchrony was associated with more frequent appearance-related victimisation, with stronger associations for girls, although patterns were also observed for boys in some analyses (Bigelow and Chaku, 2025). These findings do not suggest that puberty causes bullying; rather, they support a developmental account in which visible difference during sensitive periods can increase the risk of targeting, while outcomes still depend heavily on peer culture, adult protection and relational support.

Practical Implications: Body-based Shame and Avoidance

Appearance-related victimisation often carries heightened shame and self-consciousness. Young people may change clothing, avoid Physical Education, withdraw socially or become distressed about their bodies. Adults may misinterpret these changes as 'teenage moodiness' rather than recognising them as potential signs of appearance-focused bullying. Support often needs to include both environmental protection and careful language that avoids reinforcing shame, for example, focusing on safety and dignity rather than appearance evaluation.

School Climate and Upstream Protective factors

Why Context and Adult Response Matter

Bullying is shaped by peer ecology and adult systems. A child's stress response is more likely to remain activated when the environment is unpredictable, adults are inconsistent or disclosures do not lead to protection. In contrast, school climates that increase relational safety, fairness and adult responsiveness can reduce both bullying behaviour and its downstream impacts.

Evidence linking School Climate, Self-regulation and Bullying Involvement

Research examining school-level factors suggests that school climate and students' emotional self-regulation are meaningfully linked to bullying involvement. A structural equation modelling study reported that emotional self-regulation was negatively associated with bullying and that school climate was significantly related to bullying, with behavioural inhibition/activation systems operating as mediators in the proposed model (Loveymi and Homaei, 2024). While this design does not establish causality, it supports a practical interpretation: environments that support regulation, belonging and consistent boundaries may reduce the likelihood of bullying becoming entrenched.

Translating Climate into Practice: What Adults can Change Quickly

'School climate' can sound abstract, but it is visible in daily micro-practices. Key indicators include whether adults intervene early, whether children know how to report safely, whether supervision is present in unstructured spaces, whether staff respond consistently across incidents, and whether the school communicates clear expectations about dignity and belonging. Hotspot supervision (corridors, toilets, lunch spaces, change rooms) is often a practical priority because bullying concentrates where adult attention is low. Consistent routines also matter: predictable arrival procedures, safe classroom transitions and clear consequences for harm reduce uncertainty and therefore reduce the stress load for targeted children. Finally, climate includes how adults talk about bullying. Messages that minimise ('ignore it', 'they are just jealous') can increase shame and silence. Messages that validate and act ('we take this seriously; you are not to blame; we will protect you') increase disclosure and recovery.

Sleep and Recovery

Sleep Disruption as a Maintaining Factor

Sleep is one of the strongest regulators of emotion, attention and stress reactivity. Bullying commonly disrupts sleep through anticipatory anxiety, rumination, nighttime checking of devices or fear of the next day. Poor sleep then amplifies distress and reduces frustration tolerance, creating a cycle that makes coping harder. Because sleep is modifiable, it is an important intervention point alongside urgent steps to stop bullying and restore safety.

Signs that Stress is Becoming Entrenched

Most children who experience bullying show signs of distress. A smaller subset shows patterns that suggest stress is becoming more persistent and may require a more intensive response. Indicators include escalating school avoidance or persistent physical complaints linked to specific contexts, marked sleep disruption or nightmares, persistent hypervigilance, sustained withdrawal and loss of interest, increasing shame or hopelessness, reactive aggression or risk-taking that appears to function as protection, and reliance on digital monitoring (compulsive checking) that prevents recovery time. These indicators are not diagnostic labels. They are prompts for adults to increase protection, coordinate care and ensure the child is not managing chronic threat alone.

Recovery Time as a Measurable Goal

A useful practical concept is recovery time: the amount of time a child spends in contexts where they feel safe enough for their body to settle. Bullying reduces recovery time by extending threat across school and home (via digital channels) and by increasing anticipatory anxiety. Interventions that create protected spaces, predictable supervision and device boundaries increase recovery time. Over weeks, this can support improvements in sleep, concentration and emotional regulation, even before wider peer dynamics fully shift.

What Brain-based Language Should, and Should Not, Imply

Avoiding Determinism and Blame

Because 'the brain' carries cultural authority, it is easy for brain-based explanations to be misunderstood. Three clarifications help keep this chapter accurate and supportive. (1) Brain differences are not destiny; development remains plastic. (2) Most evidence is associative; bullying is intertwined with other factors and bidirectional pathways. (3) Some adaptations are protective in the short term (hypervigilance, avoidance, social monitoring), but become problematic when they persist after danger has passed.

Compliant Phrasing Examples for Practice

Helpful phrasing includes: 'Bullying can be associated with changes in how children respond to threat'; 'For some children, repeated victimisation may increase strain on regulation and attention'; 'These reactions are understandable in the context of stress'; and 'With safety and support, stress responses can settle and recalibrate'. Phrases to avoid include: 'Bullying damages the brain', 'This will affect them forever' or 'Their brain is broken'. Using cautious language does not minimise harm; it keeps claims accurate while maintaining hope and supporting action.

Implications for Support

What helps Stress Systems Rebalance

If bullying-related changes are best understood as stress adaptations, the foundations of support become clearer. Recovery is supported when adults reliably provide safety and predictability (clear responses and reduced exposure to those causing harm), relational protection (at least one trusted adult who listens and acts), restored belonging (structured opportunities for connection), emotion and regulation support (co-regulation, skills building and therapeutic input when needed), and sleep and recovery opportunities (routines and reduced nighttime digital exposure).

Documentation and Escalation for Professionals

For schools, this often requires moving beyond single-incident thinking: patterns need monitoring, hotspot supervision needs strengthening, and online harms require coordinated responses. For health professionals, it is important to document the bullying exposure profile, functional impacts (sleep, appetite, concentration, attendance) and risk indicators (self-harm thoughts, hopelessness, unsafe retaliation) (Van Geel et al., 2014). For parents, support frequently includes both advocacy and reassurance that the child's reactions make sense in context, alongside practical steps to rebuild competence and connection.

When Additional Support is Indicated

Some children benefit from brief, school-based support once bullying stops. Others require more sustained help, especially when distress is entrenched or when bullying intersects with prior adversity or neurodevelopmental need. Indicators for additional support include persistent sleep disruption, marked functional decline, panic symptoms, trauma-like symptoms, self-harm or significant isolation. In these cases, coordinated care is important: the child needs both psychological support and environmental protection. Therapy cannot substitute for safety. Conversely, stopping bullying without addressing entrenched shame, fear and avoidance can leave a child vulnerable to ongoing difficulties.

A Short Illustrative Formulation Example

A 13-year-old reports headaches and refuses to go to school on Mondays. The pattern emerges around a lunchtime hotspot where peers film and share humiliating clips. The young person checks their phone late at night to see whether new content has been posted, leading to poor sleep and increased anxiety. In class, they appear distracted and irritable; staff interpret this as defiance. A formulation approach reframes the behaviour as threat management: avoidance protects against humiliation; phone-checking attempts to regain certainty; irritability reflects fatigue and vigilance. Intervention targets therefore include immediate protection at the hotspot, a coordinated response to online harassment, sleep support (reducing nighttime access) and rebuilding safe belonging through structured activities and a trusted adult check-in. The aim is not to 'fix' the child's brain, but to restore safety so their stress systems can recalibrate.

Chapter Summary

Bullying can act as a chronic social stressor that repeatedly activates threat systems and reduces recovery time. For some children, particularly those who are vulnerable, unsupported or exposed over long periods, this stress can be associated with differences in the development and functioning of networks involved in threat detection, social evaluation, emotion regulation and learning. At the same time, children vary widely in their outcomes, and it is neither accurate nor helpful to describe bullying as producing inevitable, permanent brain harm.

A balanced account recognises bidirectional pathways, the distinct needs of children who are both bullied and bully others, and the protective power of timely intervention. The consistent priority across contexts is the same: stop the harm, restore safety, and ensure reliable adult protection and pathways back to belonging. The next chapter turns to recovery and resilience, focusing on how supportive relationships, safe environments and evidence-informed interventions can help stress systems settle and development re-stabilise.

Key Takeaways

- Bullying often functions like sustained threat, affecting learning and behaviour while it is active
- Careful language matters: neither minimising nor over-pathologising helps children recover
- Some vulnerabilities can increase risk, and bullying can then amplify those vulnerabilities

- Children who are bullied and bully others need a coordinated plan, not labels
- Recovery is common when safety, predictability and support become consistent

References

Arseneault, L. (2018) 'Annual research review: The persistent and pervasive impact of being bullied in childhood and adolescence', *Journal of Child Psychology and Psychiatry*, 59(4), pp. 405–421.

Arseneault, L., Bowes, L. and Shakoor, S. (2010) 'Bullying victimization in youths and mental health problems: "Much ado about nothing"?', *Psychological Medicine*, 40(5), pp. 717–729.

Balluerka, N., Aliri, J., Goñi-Balentziaga, O. and Gorostiaga, A. (2023) 'Association between bullying victimization, anxiety and depression in childhood and adolescence: The mediating effect of self-esteem', *Revista de Psicodidáctica (English ed.)*, 28(1), pp. 26–34. doi:10.1016/j.psicoe.2022.11.001.

Bigelow, J.C. and Chaku, N. (2025) 'Appearance-related victimization and pubertal asynchrony: Identifying sex-specific vulnerabilities', *Journal of Youth and Adolescence*, 54, pp. 821–836. doi:10.1007/s10964-024-02099-z.

Chen, G., Kong, Y., Deater-Deckard, K. and Zhang, W. (2018) 'Bullying victimization heightens cortisol response to psychosocial stress in Chinese children', *Journal of Abnormal Child Psychology*, 46(5), pp. 1051–1059. doi:10.1007/s10802-017-0366-6.

Domínguez, T., Nieto, L., Fresán, A., Sheinbaum, T. and Robles, R. (2025) 'The association of bullying and self-esteem with psychotic-like experiences and clinical high risk for psychosis symptoms', *Child and Adolescent Psychiatry and Mental Health*, 19(1), 51. doi:10.1186/s13034-025-00900-w.

Du Plessis, M.R., Smeekens, S., Cillessen, A.H.N., Whittle, S. and Güroğlu, B. (2019) 'Bullying the brain? Longitudinal links between childhood peer victimization, cortisol, and adolescent brain structure', *Frontiers in Psychology*, 9, 2706. doi:10.3389/fpsyg.2018.02706.

Evans-Lacko, S., Takizawa, R., Brimblecombe, N., King, D., Knapp, M., Maughan, B. and Arseneault, L. (2017) 'Childhood bullying victimization is associated with use of mental health services over five decades: A longitudinal nationally representative cohort study', *Psychological Medicine*, 47(1), pp. 127–135. doi:10.1017/S0033291716001719

Gong, X., Tian, T., Xu, J., Qin, S. and Lin, D. (2024) 'Psychophysiological factors moderate amygdala–prefrontal connectivity linked to perceived peer victimization and depressive symptoms in preadolescent migrant children', *Depression and Anxiety*, 2024(1), p. 5596651. doi:10.1155/2024/5596651.

Ke, T., De Simoni, S., Barker, E.D. and Smith, P. (2022) 'The association between peer-victimisation and structural and functional brain outcomes: A systematic review', *JCPP Advances*, 2, e12081. doi:10.1002/jcv2.12081.

Li, Y., Tian, E., Abu Bakar, Z.B. and Ashari, Z.B.M. (2025) 'Gender differences in the relationship between bullying victimization and mobile phone addiction among adolescents: The mediating roles of depression and social anxiety', *BMC Psychology*, 13, 847. doi:10.1186/s40359-025-03202-0.

Liu, M., Liu, A., Liu, S., Xu, B. and Wu, X. (2025) 'Longitudinal cross-lagged relationships of complex post-traumatic stress disorder, depression, and anxiety among adolescents and emerging adults with childhood bullying victimization experiences', *Depression and Anxiety*, 2025, 9166230. doi:10.1155/da/9166230.

Loveymi, K.D. and Homaei, R. (2024) 'Prediction of school bullying based on school climate and emotional self-regulation: The mediating role of brain-behavioural systems', *Emotional and Behavioural Difficulties*, 29(3), pp. 1–9. doi:10.1080/13632752.2024.2366111.

McEwen, B.S. (2017) 'Neurobiological and systemic effects of chronic stress', *Chronic Stress*, 1, 2470547017692328. doi: 10.1177/2470547017692328..

McLaughlin, K.A., Sheridan, M.A., Humphreys, K.L., Belsky, J. and Ellis, B.J. (2021) 'The value of dimensional models of early experience: Thinking clearly about concepts and categories', *Perspectives on Psychological Science*, 16(6), pp. 1463–1472.

McLaughlin, K.A., Sheridan, M.A. and Lambert, H.K. (2014) 'Childhood adversity and neural development: Deprivation and threat as distinct dimensions of early experience', *Neuroscience and Biobehavioral Reviews*, 47, pp. 578–591. doi: 10.1016/j.neubiorev.2014.10.012.

Menken MS, Rodriguez Rivera PJ, Isaiah A, Ernst T, Cloak CC, Chang L. (2023) 'Longitudinal alterations in brain morphometry mediated the effects of bullying victimization on cognitive development in preadolescents', *Developmental Cognitive Neuroscience*, 61, 101247. doi:10.1016/j.dcn.2023.101247.

Muetzel RL, Mulder RH, Lamballais S, Cortes Hidalgo AP, Jansen P, Güroğlu B, Vernooiji MW, Hillegers M, White T, El Marroun, H and Tiemeier, H. (2019) 'Frequent bullying involvement and brain morphology in children', *Frontiers in Psychiatry*, 10, 696. doi:10.3389/fpsyt.2019.00696.

Musci, R.J., Bettencourt, A.F., Sisto, D., Maher, B., Uhl, G., Ialongo, N. and Bradshaw, C.P. (2018) 'Evaluating the genetic susceptibility to peer reported bullying behaviors', *Psychiatry Research*, 263, pp. 193–198. doi:10.1016/j.psychres.2018.03.016.

Real-Fernández, M., Navarro-Soria, I., Rosales-Gómez, M. and Delgado, B. (2025) 'Problematic internet use and its relationship with cyberbullying, anxiety, and executive functions in adolescence', *Children*, 12(4), 503. doi:10.3390/children12040503.

Sayler, K., McLaughlin, K.A. and Belsky, J. (2025) 'Early-life threat and deprivation: Are children similarly affected by exposure to each?', *Child Development*, 96(2), pp. 606–618. doi:10.1111/cdev.14188

Schoeler, T., Choi, S.W., Dudbridge, F., Baldwin, J., Duncan, L., Cecil, C.M., Walton, E., Viding, E., McCrory, E. and Pingault, J.-B. (2019) 'Multi-polygenic score approach to identifying individual vulnerabilities associated with the risk of exposure to bullying', *JAMA Psychiatry*, 76(7), pp. 730–738. doi:10.1001/jamapsychiatry.2019.0310.

Shonkoff JP, Garner AS; Committee on Psychosocial Aspects of Child and Family Health; Committee on Early Childhood, Adoption, and Dependent Care; Section on Developmental and Behavioral Pediatrics. (2012) 'The lifelong effects of early childhood adversity and toxic stress', *Pediatrics*, 129(1), pp. e232–e246. doi: 10.1542/peds.2011-2663.

Takizawa, R., Maughan, B. and Arseneault, L. (2014) 'Adult health outcomes of childhood bullying victimization: Evidence from a five-decade longitudinal British birth cohort', *American Journal of Psychiatry*, 171(7), pp. 777–784.

Vaillancourt, T., Hymel, S. and McDougall, P. (2013) 'The biological underpinnings of peer victimization: Understanding why and how the effects of bullying can last a lifetime', *Theory Into Practice*, 52(4), pp. 241–248. doi: 10.1080/00405841.2013.829726.

Van Geel, M., Vedder, P. and Tanilon, J. (2014) 'Relationship between peer victimization, cyberbullying, and suicide in children and adolescents: A meta-analysis', *JAMA Pediatrics*, 168(5), pp. 435–442. doi: 10.1001/jamapediatrics.2013.4143.

Wade, M., Wright, L. and Finegold, K.E. (2022) 'The effects of early life adversity on children's mental health and cognitive functioning', *Translational Psychiatry*, 12, p. 244. doi: 10.1038/s41398-022-02001-0.

Wen, X., Shu, Y., Qu, D., Wang, Y., Cui, Z., Zhang, X. and Chen, R. (2023) 'Associations of bullying perpetration and peer victimization subtypes with preadolescent's suicidality, non-suicidal self-injury, neurocognition, and brain development', *BMC Medicine*, 21, p. 141. doi: 10.1186/s12916-023-02808-8.

Wolke, D., Copeland, W.E., Angold, A. and Costello, E.J. (2013) 'Impact of bullying in childhood on adult health, wealth, crime and social outcomes', *Psychological Science*, 24(10), pp. 1958–1970. doi: 10.1177/0956797613481608.

Wolke, D. and Lereya, S.T. (2015) 'Long-term effects of bullying', *Archives of Disease in Childhood*, 100(9), pp. 879–885. doi: 10.1136/archdischild-2014-306667.

Part II

Helping Children to Heal
(or Recovery and Healing)

Chapter 4

The Road to Recovery

Abstract

Recovery after bullying is possible, but it is rarely quick or uniform. When a child has been repeatedly targeted, their nervous system often adapts to threat through heightened vigilance, avoidance, emotional reactivity or withdrawal. These patterns can look fixed, especially to adults who feel helpless watching a child struggle. However, children's brains and psychological systems remain capable of recalibration across development. This chapter explains what recovery can realistically look like after chronic peer victimisation, including how stress systems settle when safety is restored, why trusted relationships matter biologically, as well as emotionally, and how evidence-based therapies support healing. It also clarifies what research supports strong, functional improvement in regulation and wellbeing, and what should be described more cautiously, such as claims about reversing specific brain-structure findings. The chapter offers practical, evidence-informed interventions for clinicians, parents and teachers, and includes a case study showing how safeguarding, relational support and therapy work together over time.

In This Chapter

- What recovery can look like (and why it is rarely quick or linear)
- How neuroplasticity really works, what is supported vs what is oversold
- The foundations of recovery: safety, stability, trust and routine
- Evidence-informed supports (school plans, therapeutic approaches, family strategies)
- Practical guidance for rebuilding confidence and belonging

Recovery is Real, But It Is Not a Straight Line

The mental health impacts of bullying described in the previous chapter highlight both the risks associated with sustained peer victimisation and the considerable potential for recovery. While repeated stress can disrupt emotional

DOI: 10.4324/9781003771777-7

wellbeing, learning and developmental trajectories, these effects are not fixed. Children's brains and psychological systems retain a strong capacity for adaptation, particularly when safety is restored and appropriate support provided.

This chapter focuses on recovery. It brings together what is known about healing following chronic peer stress, the role of relationships and therapeutic support, and the conditions under which recovery is most likely. Healing is possible, but it is not immediate, uniform or guaranteed. Progress often occurs gradually and varies according to the child's history, environment and the availability of consistent support.

For health professionals, parents and educators, it can help to hold two truths at once:

- Many children make significant gains when bullying stops and support becomes reliable.
- Some children need longer and more structured intervention, especially when bullying has occurred alongside earlier adversity, neurodevelopmental vulnerabilities or ongoing stress at home or at school.

Recovery is not a single event. It is a process of rebuilding safety, restoring regulation and supporting the child to reconnect with learning, peers and a sense of self that is not defined by what happened to them.

Scope and Support Note

This chapter is designed to support understanding and informed decision-making for parents, teachers and non-specialist professionals. It does not provide diagnosis or individual clinical treatment advice. Where children show high levels of distress or risk (for example, self-harm, suicidal thoughts or persistent trauma-like symptoms), readers should follow local safeguarding procedures and seek assessment from appropriately qualified professionals.

How the Brain Can Heal after Bullying

As discussed in Chapter 2 and Chapter 3, repeated peer victimisation can train the stress system to anticipate threat, shaping attention, sleep, behaviour and emotional reactivity. In recovery, the key question becomes: what helps the system learn safety again?

Across developmental neuroscience, psychology and trauma research, the brain remains adaptable throughout childhood, adolescence and into adulthood. This capacity for change is referred to as neural plasticity: the ability of neural systems to reorganise in response to experience.

Plasticity does not mean a simple 'reset' after adversity. More often, it looks like gradual recalibration under safer conditions, new patterns of regulation, learning and emotional response becoming more available when stress is reduced and supportive conditions are established (Gee and Cohodes, 2023; Gunnar, 2020).

It is also important to be precise about what can be claimed. Evidence most strongly supports functional improvement, for example, improved regulation, reduced anxiety and better day-to-day coping, when safety and support are sustained. Claims about reversing specific structural brain differences are less certain and should not be promised for an individual child (Sonuga-Barke, 2017).

What is Neural Plasticity, and What Does It Realistically Mean for Recovery?

A simple analogy can be useful here. Think of the brain as a network of roads. When a child has been repeatedly targeted, 'threat routes' may become the quickest and most automatic pathways. The child may appear on edge, avoidant, reactive or shut down, not because they are choosing these responses, but because their system has learned that social settings are unsafe.

With safety and support, the brain can begin to build alternative routes: pathways associated with calm, problem-solving, social approach and self-trust. That is plasticity in action. At the same time, plasticity does not guarantee a uniform outcome. Children with prolonged adversity, multiple stressors, neurodevelopmental differences or limited support may require longer and more intensive intervention. Recovery is best understood as a process, not a single event, and setbacks are common (Gunnar, 2020; Gee and Cohodes, 2023).

Probable versus Speculative: Making An Evidence-based Distinction

Because 'brain' explanations can be compelling, it is worth keeping language anchored in what research supports most clearly.

Probable (strongly supported across child development and stress research):

- When bullying stops and safety becomes reliable, many children show gradual improvements in sleep, attention, emotion regulation and confidence.
- Trusted adults support recovery by reducing stress reactivity and strengthening regulation over time.
- Evidence-based therapies can reduce anxiety, depression and trauma-like symptoms, and improve coping and functioning.

More speculative (important research areas, but not something to promise):

- Structural brain findings observed in group-level studies will 'reverse' in a clear, predictable way for any individual child.
- Recovery follows one timeline or one pathway.
- Removing bullying alone is sufficient for recovery in every case.

This is not pessimistic. It is honest, and it helps families stay engaged when progress is slow or uneven.

How Recovery Happens

Recovery is most likely when three conditions come together:

1. The stressor is reduced or removed (bullying ends; risk is actively managed).
2. The child is supported by consistent, trusted adults (home and school).
3. Skills and meaning-making are supported (through therapy, coaching or structured emotional support).

This matters because therapy cannot substitute for safety. A child cannot settle in a system that continues to be activated by repeated peer harm. In practice, the most effective recovery plans are blended: safeguarding plus relational support plus targeted intervention.

Foundations of Recovery: Safety and Stability

Establishing Safety First

Recovery is difficult to sustain unless a child feels safe, physically, emotionally and socially. In practice, this means more than the absence of incidents on record. It means a child can move through the day without anticipating harm, humiliation or exclusion

For parents and teachers, the key question is therefore not only, *'Has the bullying stopped?'* but also, *'Does the child experience it as having stopped?'* After repeated targeting, many children remain watchful, even when adults have intervened. That expectation of threat can continue to drive anxiety, avoidance and heightened reactivity.

This is why reassurance on its own is rarely enough. Safety often needs to be made visible and predictable, so the child can test it repeatedly. Helpful measures may include:

- A named adult the child can go to immediately
- Planned check-ins (more frequent at first, then reduced as confidence grows)

- Agreed safe routes and safe spaces
- Supported transitions (arrival, corridors, lunch, dismissal)
- Careful management of higher-risk contexts, without isolating the child socially
- Online safety steps (blocking and reporting, evidence capture where appropriate, and clear adult oversight)

At home, consistent caregiving, emotional availability and reassurance help stabilise stress systems and support emotional recovery. When adults remain calm and predictable, children receive the repeated message: 'You are not alone with this.'

Supportive Adult Relationships

Stable, caring adults are central to recovery. This may be a parent, teacher, therapist, learning mentor, coach or another trusted adult. Children who feel believed and understood are more likely to regain confidence, re-engage with learning and take small risks in social settings again.

Relational support is not simply 'being nice'. It is the everyday process of helping a child regulate. A calm adult response can reduce the intensity of distress in the moment and, over time, support the child to develop more reliable self-regulation. For many children, recovery is built through repeated experiences of being heard, being protected and being responded to consistently.

In school settings, these relational foundations work best when safeguarding practices are clear and dependable. Trauma-informed and restorative approaches can be helpful when implemented carefully and when they do not place pressure on the child to reconcile or 'move on' before they feel safe. The priority remains safety, accountability and restoring the child's sense of agency.

Turning the Recovery Triangle into a Plan: What Changes in the First 6–12 Weeks

For many children, the first phase of recovery is less about insight and more about predictability. Adults sometimes expect the child to 'feel better' once an incident is addressed, but threat-learning does not switch off instantly. A useful way to think about early recovery is as a sequence of *small, repeated safety experiences* that gradually outweigh the child's expectation of harm (Gunnar, 2020; Gee and Cohodes, 2023).

What follows is not a clinical protocol. It is a practical scaffold that schools, parents and non-specialist professionals can adapt in partnership with appropriately qualified clinicians where needed.

Weeks 1–2: stabilisation and visible safety

In the early stage, the priority is to reduce the child's exposure to threat cues and make adult protection *predictable*. For schools, this often means moving from general reassurance ('Tell us if anything happens') to an explicit plan the child can rely on. This might include a named adult, planned check-ins and clear supervision during high-risk times (arrival, corridors, lunch, dismissal). For parents, it often means keeping mornings calm and structured, and reducing repeated questioning that can unintentionally keep the child in 'reliving' mode.

A helpful marker of stabilisation is not whether the child is cheerful, but whether the day becomes *more manageable*: fewer tears at the door, fewer somatic complaints, less escalation after school or a small improvement in sleep (Gunnar, 2020).

Weeks 3–6: supported re-engagement

Once the child is not in constant escalation, the next task is to rebuild participation. Avoidance is understandable and protective in the short term, but if it becomes entrenched, it can shrink the child's world and maintain fear. Many children benefit from a gradual return plan that protects dignity and reduces repeated exposure to high-risk contexts while the system relearns safety (Arseneault, 2018).

In school, supported re-engagement may involve:

- Partial timetables that increase gradually
- Supported entry points (arriving slightly early, meeting a trusted adult)
- Planned transitions with supervision
- Careful groupings for partner and group work
- Short 'reset' options without punishment when overwhelmed

At home, it often involves rebuilding one safe routine at a time: sleep, food, movement, then social activity. The goal is not to push the child back into the deep end; it is to help them have success experiences that contradict the belief 'I can't cope'.

Weeks 6–12: belonging and confidence-building

For longer-term recovery, belonging is not optional. Bullying is social harm: it attacks the child's standing, identity and safety within a group. This is why recovery plans that focus only on individual coping skills can leave children technically 'safe', but still socially stranded.

Schools can support belonging through structured roles that do not depend on popularity: clubs, interest groups, responsibilities, mentoring schemes, protected peer partnerships or small-group projects with adults actively shaping the culture. For some children, a single consistent place to belong each week has more impact than multiple one-off initiatives (Gee and Cohodes, 2023).

For adolescents, belonging must be real rather than symbolic. If bullying was identity-based (race, disability, sexuality, gender expression, religion), recovery is strengthened when the school response includes visible inclusion and anti-discrimination action, not only individual support for the targeted young person (Department for Education, 2024).

A note on pace

The timeline above is not a promise. It is a guide. Some children stabilise quickly once protection is consistent; others take longer, particularly where there has been earlier adversity, ongoing stress or neurodevelopmental vulnerabilities. In these cases, progress is often uneven. The most important thing is that adults interpret slower progress as a signal to strengthen the system, not as a reason to withdraw support (Sonuga-Barke, 2017; Gunnar, 2020).

Evidence-based Psychological Interventions

A range of interventions are associated with improvements in anxiety, low mood, trauma-like symptoms and coping following experiences of peer victimisation. Choice of approach should be guided by the child's age and developmental stage, presenting difficulties, neurodevelopmental needs, family context and what is realistically available. Access and timing also matter: some children can engage with structured therapeutic work quickly; others first need safety and stabilisation.

The aim is not to 'treat bullying' as a single issue, but to support recovery from its effects: anxiety, low mood, trauma-like symptoms, avoidance, shame, dysregulation and disrupted self-concept.

Cognitive Behavioural Therapy (CBT), including Trauma-focused CBT (TF-CBT)

Cognitive behavioural therapy (CBT) helps children identify and challenge unhelpful thought patterns and replace them with more balanced and compassionate interpretations. It also teaches coping strategies such as relaxation, graded exposure to feared settings, problem-solving and behavioural activation (rebuilding activities that support mood and confidence) (Arseneault, 2018; Lydecker, 2022).

For many bullied children, this approach is helpful because bullying often leaves behind strong beliefs such as:

- 'I'm not safe.'
- 'People will always turn on me.'
- 'If I speak up, it gets worse.'
- 'It must be my fault.'
- 'I'm weak/disgusting/unlikable.'

CBT supports children to recognise these beliefs as understandable responses to harm, while also helping them test new interpretations and build new behavioural experiences.

For some children, bullying has created trauma-like symptoms: intrusive memories, panic responses in specific places, nightmares, shutdown and persistent avoidance. In these cases, trauma-focused CBT (TF-CBT) is particularly relevant because it is designed for repeated threat, and includes structured work on regulation skills, processing distressing experiences and reducing shame. TF-CBT also often involves caregivers, which can be an important protective factor in recovery (Lydecker, 2022).

In practical terms, TF-CBT can be adapted to bullying contexts by incorporating:

- A clear safety plan alongside school involvement
- Work on self-blame and shame
- Careful processing of 'hot spots' (worst moments, humiliation, betrayal by peers)
- Rebuilding a sense of personal agency and social confidence
- Strategies for triggers linked to school spaces or online cues

Eye Movement Desensitisation and Reprocessing (EMDR)

Eye movement desensitisation and reprocessing (EMDR) is increasingly used with children who have experienced interpersonal stress. It supports the processing of distressing memories and reduces emotional reactivity linked to those memories (Barron et al., 2019).

Most evidence for EMDR in young people relates to trauma and post-traumatic stress disorder (PTSD) presentations rather than bullying-specific clinical trials. However, it can be helpful when bullying experiences have become emotionally overwhelming or intrusive, particularly when the child feels stuck, reliving events, panicking in specific contexts or feeling flooded by shame.

EMDR is typically delivered by trained clinicians. It is not a stand-alone solution: it works best alongside ongoing safeguarding and stability. If the bullying continues, or if the child remains exposed to ongoing threat, memory processing work is often less effective and may feel destabilising.

Mindfulness and Relaxation Skills

Mindfulness-based skills can help children notice what is happening inside them (their thoughts, sensations and emotions) without being immediately swept away by it. In simple terms, mindfulness builds the ability to pause.

For bullied children, this can be especially helpful for:

- Panic sensations and body-based anxiety
- Shame spirals
- Anger surges and impulsive reactions
- Sleep difficulties

Practical tools that suit children and adolescents include:

- Paced breathing
- Grounding exercises
- Short body scans
- Emotion labelling
- Brief guided audio exercises (2–5 minutes)

Mindfulness should be introduced carefully. Some children find internal focus uncomfortable at first, especially if they have strong anxiety or trauma-like symptoms. In these cases, grounding through movement may be a better starting point.

Creative Expression and Play-based Approaches

Some children cannot easily talk about what happened, or they do not yet have words for the mix of fear, humiliation, anger and loss that bullying can create. Creative approaches can support expression without forcing disclosure before the child is ready.
Examples include:

- Art-based expression (drawings, comics, collage)
- Drama and role play
- Music and rhythm
- Narrative work

Exercise, Movement and Physical Health

Regular physical activity supports mood, sleep and stress regulation. For bullied children, movement can also be a pathway back to a sense of competence and identity, particularly when confidence has been damaged.

The goal is not performance. It is regulation, routine and positive experience. Options include:

- Walking outdoors with a trusted adult
- Swimming

- Dance or martial arts
- Team sport (when safe and supportive)
- Yoga or structured stretching

Some children avoid sport because bullying has occurred in change rooms or team settings. In those cases, begin with safe, predictable forms of movement and gradually rebuild.

Peer Support and Group Interventions

Support groups or therapeutic groups can reduce isolation and shame. Hearing 'it happened to me too' can be powerfully regulating. Groups can also teach practical coping skills and social confidence.

Group work is not suitable for every child. It works best:

- When the child is not currently at high risk of re-victimisation within the group
- When confidentiality and safety are strong
- When the group has clear structure and skilled facilitation
- When participation is voluntary and paced

Family Involvement and Education

Families play a crucial role in healing. Educating parents and siblings about the impact of bullying and involving them in the recovery process helps create a nurturing and consistent support system. (Gee and Cohodes, 2023).

Practical family-level recovery steps include:

- Keeping routines stable (sleep, meals, school mornings)
- Reducing over-questioning (which can feel like pressure)
- Responding to distress with validation and calm action
- Helping the child re-engage with safe activities
- Coordinating with the school in a clear, documented way
- Monitoring online spaces without shaming or punishing the child

Family counselling can be helpful when bullying has created ongoing conflict at home or when parents disagree on how to respond to it.

Intervention Map: Matching Needs to Support

The aim is not to match every child to a single 'perfect' intervention, but to choose support that fits the main difficulty at that point in time, and to review it as the child stabilises. The map below can be used as a shared language for clinicians, parents and schools when coordinating support. It is intended as evidence-informed signposting, not as a substitute for individual assessment (Table 4.1).

Support works best when combined. Skills and therapy are most effective when safety is real and belonging is actively rebuilt.

Table 4.1 Intervention map: symptom focus and best-fit support

Presenting difficulty	*What may be driving it*	*Best-fit support (examples)*
Generalised anxiety, worry, anticipatory fear	Ongoing expectation of threat; hypervigilance	CBT (including graded re-engagement with feared situations) plus a visible school safety plan
Intrusive memories, nightmares, panic triggers	Trauma-like stress responses; cue reactivity	TF-CBT and/or EMDR where safeguarding and stability are in place
Severe school avoidance/refusal	Conditioned fear; loss of felt safety; overwhelm	Coordinated graded return plan plus CBT; short-term adjustments while re-entry is rebuilt
Emotional dysregulation (anger surges, shutdown)	Overloaded regulation system; low window of tolerance	Skills-based work (informed by CBT- or dialectical behaviour therapy (DBT)), plus adult co-regulation coaching and predictable routines
Social withdrawal, isolation, loss of belonging	Shame, mistrust, social threat sensitivity	Structured belonging (club/role/responsibility) plus gradual social re-engagement; group work only when safe
Low mood, loss of pleasure, hopelessness	Reduced reinforcement; internalised negative beliefs	CBT behavioural activation plus supportive activity scheduling; consider GP/CAMHS assessment if severe or persistent
Shame-based self-beliefs and self-blame	Internalised meaning-making ('It's my fault')	Cognitive restructuring plus narrative work; compassion-focused elements where appropriate
Family tension, conflict, over-protection	Stress spillover; accommodation patterns	Parental guidance; family therapy where available; consistent routines and calm, unified messaging
Identity-related distress (race, disability, LGBTQ+ targeting)	Minority stress; threat + invalidation	Affirmative practice plus safe peer connection; ensure clear anti-discrimination action in school

Clarifying Expectations: What Recovery Often Looks like in Real Life

It is tempting to look for a clear 'end point' after bullying; proof that the child is fine again. In reality, recovery is usually piecemeal. Early signs tend to be small shifts in the child's body and daily functioning before confidence fully returns. These may include:

- Fewer stomach aches or headaches before school
- More willingness to enter school with support
- Less scanning and checking behaviours
- Improved sleep or fewer nightmares
- A reduction in angry outbursts or tearfulness
- A gradual return of humour, curiosity or appetite
- Tentative steps back into friendships
- More stable concentration in lessons

Setbacks are common, particularly around anniversaries, school transitions, exams or renewed contact with peers involved in bullying. A setback does not mean failure. It often means a trigger has activated the old threat expectation. The recovery task is to respond early, restoring safety cues, strengthening connection with trusted adults, and re-establishing regulation supports, rather than waiting for things to escalate.

When Recovery Stalls: Red Flags and When to Refer

Recovery is often uneven. Many children show gradual improvement once bullying stops and adults respond consistently. However, there are times when distress remains high or increases despite reasonable safeguarding and support. This section offers evidence-informed signposting. It is not a substitute for clinical assessment, diagnosis or crisis care (Department for Education, 2024).

For child and adolescent mental health services (CAMHS) and safeguarding professionals, it can be useful to consider three questions:

1. Is there immediate risk?
2. Has there been a marked drop in functioning?
3. Are there persistent trauma-like symptoms or complex presentations that warrant specialist assessment?

Where risk is suspected, follow your setting's safeguarding policy and local referral pathways (Department for Education, 2024).

If Immediate Risk is Suspected

Seek urgent assessment and follow local safeguarding and crisis procedures if any of the following are present (National Institute for Health and Care Excellence, 2022; Department for Education, 2024):

- Suicidal thoughts, plans or statements of wanting to die, including indirect or ambiguous disclosures (National Institute for Health and Care Excellence, 2022).
- Self-harm behaviours, escalating risk-taking or rapid deterioration in mood (National Institute for Health and Care Excellence, 2022).
- Disclosure of ongoing abuse, exploitation or serious threats linked to the bullying (including coercion, sharing of images, blackmail or threats of violence) (Department for Education, 2024).

If Symptoms are Severe or Persistent: Consider Specialist Assessment

Consider specialist assessment (for example CAMHS or equivalent services) when symptoms are persistent, severe or significantly impair day-to-day functioning. Indicators can include (National Institute for Health and Care Excellence, 2018; National Institute for Health and Care Excellence, 2019; National Institute for Health and Care Excellence, 2022):

- Severe or persistent school refusal (weeks rather than days), especially when linked to panic symptoms, vomiting, shutdown or marked distress on approach to school (National Institute for Health and Care Excellence, 2019).
- Trauma-like symptoms that persist (intrusive memories, nightmares, intense trigger reactions, avoidance, startling, emotional numbing) (National Institute for Health and Care Excellence, 2018).
- Significant changes in eating, weight or body image, particularly when the bullying targeted appearance, disability, gender expression or identity (National Institute for Health and Care Excellence, 2019).
- Persistent dissociation, 'zoning out', or shutdown that interferes with learning and relationships (National Institute for Health and Care Excellence, 2018).
- Marked functional decline (sleep disruption, inability to concentrate, withdrawal from activities, loss of previously stable friendships) (National Institute for Health and Care Excellence, 2019).
- Substance use, risky online behaviour, or sexualised risk linked to coercion or social pressure (Department for Education, 2024)

Clinical Note: What 'Stalled' Recovery Can Mean

Stalled recovery does not mean a child is choosing not to get better. It often means the nervous system is still operating as if threat is present. This can happen when the child continues to encounter reminders (corridors, online cues, friendship groups), when shame has become entrenched, or when there are additional stressors at home or in the wider peer context (National Institute for Health and Care Excellence, 2018; Department for Education, 2024).

A useful approach is to review three domains together. (1) Is safety genuinely in place? (2) Does the child have at least one reliable regulating adult connection? (3) Are evidence-based skills and therapeutic support being offered at the right pace? When one domain is missing, progress is often slower.

In all cases, documentation helps. Record concerns, actions taken and the child's current level of functioning. This supports continuity of care and clear safeguarding decision-making (Department for Education, 2024).

Box 4.1 Recovery After Complex Trauma and Bullying

Leah, 11, had experienced multiple stressors before the bullying began. Her early life included family instability and frequent moves. She had learned to be 'on alert' and was sensitive to rejection. When she started a new school, a small group of peers began targeting her. The bullying was both in-person and online. It included name-calling, exclusion, sharing photos without permission and threats about what would happen if she told an adult.

At home, Leah became irritable and withdrawn. She stopped asking to see friends. Mornings became a battleground. She reported stomach pain and asked repeatedly to stay home from school. At night she struggled to settle and began sleeping with the light on. She also became highly reactive to small comments from family members, snapping, then crying and apologising, and then shutting down.

Stage 1: Stabilisation and safety. The first priority was to stop the bullying and reduce Leah's daily exposure to threat cues. The school implemented a safety plan with a named staff contact, supervised transitions, monitored seating arrangements and a clear response protocol if incidents occurred. Her parents were supported to respond consistently: calm reassurance, reduced pressure to 'explain everything' and predictable routines.

Stage 2: Regulation and processing. Leah began therapy focused on anxiety and trauma-like symptoms. Early sessions emphasised regulation: breathing practices, grounding and identifying triggers. Only once she could settle more reliably did therapy move towards processing key bullying moments and working on shame-based beliefs.

Stage 3: Reconnection and growth. As symptoms reduced, Leah gradually re-engaged with safe activities. She joined a small lunchtime club with a supportive teacher, which gave her a peer setting structured around shared interest rather than social status. She began a movement-based hobby outside school, which rebuilt her confidence and gave her body a sense of competence. The school continued check-ins, then slowly reduced them as Leah's confidence grew.

What helped most: bullying was actively addressed (not minimised); adults acted consistently and predictably; therapy was paced (regulation first, processing later); shame beliefs were named and reframed gently; reconnection was structured through safe activities.

Box 4.2 Cyberbullying and Identity-based Targeting in Adolescence

Aisha is 15. Over the course of a year, she was subjected to repeated online harassment linked to her race and her sexual orientation. Anonymous accounts circulated edited images of her and encouraged others to exclude her socially. The bullying did not occur only at school. It followed her home through her phone.

When the school intervened and the accounts were removed, staff expected an improvement. Instead, Aisha became increasingly withdrawn. She avoided group work, reported feeling watched and described difficulty sleeping. Her grades declined. She did not describe herself as 'traumatised'. She described herself as 'exhausted'.

Assessment suggested ongoing hypervigilance and intrusive rumination. Aisha reported repeatedly checking social media to see whether new content had appeared. She struggled with trust, particularly in peer relationships, and avoided settings where peers might take photographs.

Recovery involved three coordinated strands: (1) clear digital safeguarding steps and predictable school responses; (2) therapy focused on shame, intrusive thoughts and safety cues; and (3) reconnection with a safe peer group that supported identity and belonging. Sleep stabilised first. Social confidence followed more slowly. What helped Aisha most was not therapy alone, but therapy alongside visible safety and real belonging.

Healing the Brain Through Connection

Positive relationships and safe environments are not simply comforting; they shape recovery. Children regulate through relationships. A calm, attuned adult can lower the intensity of a child's distress, help them name what is happening, and offer practical steps that restore a sense of control.

For children recovering from bullying, connection supports:

- Confidence building
- Re-learning trust
- Managing stress and big emotions
- Feeling safe in group settings

These needs are real and deserve compassion and commitment from adults. The aim is not to erase what happened, but to help the child move forward without carrying a constant threat in their body and mind.

Recovery in Schools: Safety, Belonging and Phased Reintegration

Schools are not only places where bullying occurs; they are also central environments for recovery. Because peer relationships and social evaluation are developmentally significant across childhood and adolescence, school-based experiences can either reinforce threat or support recalibration. When safety, belonging and structured reintegration are prioritised, school becomes part of the healing process rather than a continuing source of stress (Gee and Cohodes, 2023; Gunnar, 2020).

A useful framework for educators is to think in three overlapping phases: immediate stabilisation, supported reintegration and confidence-building through belonging. These phases are not rigid stages. Some children move quickly between them; others need more time in each area. The purpose of the framework is not to label children, but to guide coordinated action.

Immediate stabilisation focuses on reducing exposure to threat cues and making safety visible. It is not enough for adults to know that a plan exists; the child must also experience that plan as real and reliable.

This may include clear supervision plans during high-risk times (arrival, corridors, lunch, dismissal), structured transitions, a named adult available without question, a rapid and predictable response to concerns, monitored seating arrangements and attention to online spillover. Safety plans should be shared in age-appropriate ways with the child so that they understand what is in place and what will happen if something goes wrong. Perceived safety is as important as objective safety in reducing stress reactivity (Gunnar, 2020).

Supported reintegration involves gradually rebuilding participation in learning and peer settings. Avoidance is a common response to bullying. However, when avoidance becomes entrenched, it can maintain anxiety and reduce opportunities for corrective social experiences. Predictable and supported exposure to feared contexts, at a pace the child can tolerate, reduces avoidance and rebuilds confidence over time (Arseneault, 2018). In practice, this may involve partial timetables that increase gradually, supervised small-group work, structured partner tasks with carefully selected peers, and supported return to previously avoided spaces.

Belonging is often the most powerful long-term protective factor. Bullying frequently damages identity and social confidence. Structured opportunities to experience acceptance in low-risk contexts can counter this. Interest-based clubs, responsibility roles, creative groups and small consistent peer groupings can provide a pathway back into connection. Developmental systems research emphasises that resilience emerges when supportive relationships and meaningful roles are available within everyday environments (Gee and Cohodes, 2023).

For adolescents in particular, identity becomes central. Where bullying has targeted race, disability, appearance, sexuality or other aspects of identity, recovery requires more than individual coping strategies. Schools must actively reinforce anti-discrimination policies and visibly support inclusion. A consistent whole-school stance reduces the likelihood that shame becomes internalised (Department for Education, 2024).

Coordination between home and school strengthens recovery. Mixed messages can inadvertently increase anxiety. Agreed language about progress, shared documentation of actions and concerns, and regular review points help reduce misunderstanding and support consistency.

Academic recovery may lag behind emotional recovery. Concentration, memory and motivation can take time to stabilise following prolonged stress. Temporary adjustments in workload or assessment expectations may therefore be appropriate, provided they are reviewed regularly and aim towards full reintegration rather than long-term withdrawal.

Finally, recovery plans should include scheduled check-ins. What feels sufficient in the first weeks after bullying stops may need adaptation later, particularly around transitions, exams or renewed online contact. Early response to setbacks prevents escalation.

Taken together, school-based recovery is most effective when it combines safeguarding clarity, relational consistency and structured opportunities for belonging. These elements align with broader developmental research demonstrating that children adapt most successfully when threat is reduced and supportive systems are strengthened (Gunnar, 2020; Gee and Cohodes, 2023).

Safeguarding and Coordination in Practice: What Helps Systems Hold Recovery

One of the reasons recovery can stall is that support is present, but fragmented. Parents may assume the school is managing the risk; the school may assume the family has secured clinical help; clinicians may not have a clear picture of what is happening from day to day. Children experience these gaps as uncertainty, and uncertainty keeps threat expectations alive.

The purpose of coordination is not paperwork for its own sake. It is to make adult protection reliable, and to reduce the number of times a child has to 'start again', explaining what happened.

1. Make safety plans concrete and shared
A safety plan is most effective when the child and the key adults understand the same basics:

- Who the child goes to first
- What happens if an incident occurs
- Where the child can go to settle without punishment
- Which settings are higher risk and how supervision is managed
- What steps are being taken online (where relevant)

For some schools, this is best held as a short, practical document that is reviewed at set intervals, with the child's voice included in age-appropriate form. Clarity also supports staff consistency, which is a protective factor in itself.

2. Document patterns, not only incidents
When bullying has been prolonged, focusing only on discrete 'incidents' can miss what the child is actually living through: cumulative exclusion, repeated humiliation and ongoing social threat. Pattern-based documentation helps safeguarding teams and clinicians to see the full picture and is often more informative than a list of isolated events.

This matters especially when harm involves coercion, image-based abuse or threats of retaliation. In those contexts, children may disclose gradually, and careful recording supports appropriate escalation through local pathways (Department for Education, 2024).

3. Use functional impact as a trigger for review
Schools and families sometimes wait for a new incident before re-opening safeguarding action. A more protective approach is to treat *functional decline* as a trigger for review: rising school avoidance, falling concentration, loss of previously stable friendships, deterioration in sleep or marked withdrawal. These shifts do not 'prove' that bullying is continuing, but do suggest that the

child is not yet experiencing safety, and that the plan needs strengthening (National Institute for Health and Care Excellence, 2018; National Institute for Health and Care Excellence, 2019).

4. Avoid inadvertent practices that increase shame
Certain well-intended responses can unintentionally reinforce humiliation or self-blame. Examples include:

- Repeated requests for the child to retell events to multiple adults
- Public or performative 'restorative' meetings that the child experiences as unsafe
- Pressuring a child to accept apologies or resume friendships
- Minimising identity-based harm ('try not to take it personally')
- Focusing on the child's coping style rather than the peer behaviour and school culture

A trauma-informed stance does not mean lowering boundaries for harmful behaviour. It means ensuring the response is predictable, protective and does not place the burden of repair on the child who was harmed.

5. Plan for online spillover
When bullying involves online spaces, 'stopping' it is often more complex than removing one account. Young people may continue checking platforms, scanning for new content, or fearing screenshots that reappear months later. A practical response combines:

- Clear reporting and evidence capture steps (where appropriate)
- Adult oversight of device use without punitive shaming
- School-based action where online behaviour intersects with peer relationships
- Attention to peer group dynamics (who is amplifying, sharing, liking)

This is also a setting where anxiety can look like 'choice' ('just stop going online'). In reality, compulsive checking often reflects threat monitoring. Supporting the young person to reduce checking typically works best when safety and belonging are also being addressed, not as a stand-alone instruction.

6. Know when to escalate
The existing 'When recovery stalls' section already signposts key thresholds. It is worth adding one additional emphasis for safeguarding and CAMHS readers: escalation decisions are often about risk plus context, not about a single symptom. Where risk is present, follow local crisis procedures (National Institute for Health and Care Excellence, 2022; Department for Education,

2024). Where risk is not immediate, but functioning is declining, early referral and coordinated planning can prevent longer-term entrenchment (National Institute for Health and Care Excellence, 2018; National Institute for Health and Care Excellence, 2019).

7. Keep the child's agency central
Bullying reduces agency. Recovery restores it. Even when adults must act decisively, children do better when they know what is happening, what the options are, and what they can do if fear spikes in the moment. Small agency support measures include:

- Agreeing on a discreet signal the child can use to leave a situation
- Giving a choice on how check-ins happen (time, place, frequency)
- Involving the child in selecting a safe club/role rather than assigning one
- Ensuring the child is not surprised by meetings or decisions that affect them

Agency is not a 'nice extra'. It is one of the mechanisms by which the system learns safety again (Gunnar, 2020; Gee and Cohodes, 2023).

8. A brief reality check for adults
Adults often feel pressure to produce a quick outcome: the bullying is addressed, the plan is written, the child should now be 'back to normal'. The reality is that recovery often lags behind resolution. That lag is not a failure of the child; it is the expected after-effect of prolonged peer threat. Systems that stay consistent through this phase, rather than withdrawing support once the headline problem appears 'solved', are the systems most likely to see confidence return over time (Sonuga-Barke, 2017; Arseneault, 2018).

Developmental Differences in Recovery: What Changes Across Childhood and Adolescence

Recovery does not look the same at every age. Bullying interacts with developmental stage, brain maturation, identity formation and social expectations. Understanding these differences helps adults respond proportionately and realistically.

A five-year-old who is excluded from play, an 11-year-old who is humiliated in front of peers, and a 15-year-old who is targeted online are not experiencing the same developmental task. Their nervous systems, cognitive capacities and social priorities differ. So too does the shape of their recovery.

Early childhood and early primary years are characterised by high reliance on co-regulation. Children may not have the language to describe what has happened, so distress often shows up behaviourally: increased clinginess, regression, irritability, somatic complaints or sudden avoidance. Consistent routines, rapid protection and stable caregiving can support the recalibration of stress responses (Gunnar, 2020).

In the late primary years, social comparison becomes more salient. Children are more likely to replay incidents, anticipate humiliation and develop self-beliefs that are shaped by rejection. At this stage, combining relational safety with developmentally appropriate cognitive support can be helpful, and structured belonging becomes increasingly protective (Arseneault, 2018; Gee and Cohodes, 2023).

Adolescence adds complexity. Puberty heightens sensitivity to peer evaluation and status. Where bullying targets identity (race, disability, sexuality, gender expression or appearance), shame can become deeply embedded and may be reinforced by wider social stigma. Cyberbullying can be persistent and difficult to escape, blurring the boundary between school and home. Recovery often requires visible safety, collaborative planning that respects autonomy, and genuine belonging (Department for Education, 2024).

Neurodevelopmental differences can shape risk and recovery. Children with autism or attention-deficit/hyperactivity disorder (ADHD) may experience bullying at higher rates and may find social threat cues harder to interpret or generalise across contexts. Recovery may require more explicit plans, predictable adult support and tailored social scaffolding.

Across stages, three principles remain consistent: safety must be reliable, at least one stable regulating adult relationship is protective, and belonging and competence rebuild identity more effectively than reassurance alone (Gee and Cohodes, 2023; Gunnar, 2020).

Complex Trajectories: Cumulative Adversity, Bully-victims and Long-term Outcomes

Not all children who are bullied follow the same recovery pathway. For some, bullying is a discrete period of harm within an otherwise stable developmental context. For others, it intersects with earlier adversity, neurodevelopmental vulnerability, or ongoing stress. In these cases, recovery can be slower, more uneven and more complex.

Research in developmental psychopathology shows that stress exposure can accumulate. Where early instability or ongoing adversity is present, bullying may add another layer of threat. This does not mean permanent damage, but it may change the baseline from which recovery begins. Group-level research links chronic stress exposure with differences in stress-related systems, yet these findings do not allow the prediction of individual destiny. Functional improvement with safety and support remains common (Sonuga-Barke, 2017; Gunnar, 2020).

Some children are both victims and perpetrators at different times. This 'bully-victim' pattern is often associated with higher dysregulation and greater social difficulty. These children benefit from approaches that combine clear boundaries and accountability with support for underlying distress and skills-building.

One of the more enduring impacts of bullying can be shame. Children may internalise narratives such as 'I am the kind of person who gets picked on'. Recovery often involves rebuilding identity through consistent acceptance, competence experiences and supportive meaning-making. Where bullying targets identity, visible institutional inclusion matters; neutrality can be experienced as silence (Department for Education, 2024).

Longitudinal research suggests that persistent peer victimisation is associated with an elevated risk of later anxiety, depression and social difficulties. However, association is not inevitability. Trajectories shift when protective systems are strengthened, particularly stable adult relationships, school connectedness and opportunities for belonging and competence (Arseneault, 2018; Gee and Cohodes, 2023).

As throughout this chapter, it is important to separate what is probable from what is speculative. It is well supported that stress systems can recalibrate when safety and support are sustained, and that coping and regulation can improve with practice and co-regulation. It is less defensible to promise uniform 'brain rewiring' or predictable structural change. Recovery is shaped by context and consistency, not a single intervention.

Practical Guidance: What to Do This Week

For Parents

- Keep school mornings predictable (same steps, calm tone, short sentences).
- Validate feelings without pushing for detail ('I believe you. I'm here. We have a plan.').
- Make sure your child knows exactly who their safe adult is at school.
- Rebuild one safe activity (small, structured, interest-based).
- Reduce shame language, even unintentionally ('Why didn't you…?' 'You have to be stronger…').
- Track sleep and appetite gently; these are often early markers of improvement.

For Teachers and School Staff

- Check in briefly and consistently (predictability matters more than long conversations).
- Protect transitions (corridors, lunch, arrival/dismissal) where bullying often happens.
- Make safety plans visible to the child (not just in staff emails).
- Use seating, grouping and supervision strategically.

- Avoid pressuring the child to 'be friends again'.
- Identify one structured belonging point (club, role, responsibility) that supports reconnection.

Closing Reflection

Recovery after bullying is possible. It is also shaped by context. When children are protected from ongoing harm, supported by steady adults and offered evidence-based interventions when needed, many regain confidence, emotional stability and learning readiness. Some recover quickly; others take longer. Both trajectories are valid.

What matters most is that adults do not confuse time passing with healing. Healing is supported by action: creating safety, strengthening relationships and giving children tools to understand their experience without being defined by it.

Key Takeaways

- Recovery is real, but it often comes in phases with setbacks
- Safeguarding and reduced exposure to threat come first
- Relationships are biological, as well as emotional protection
- Therapy works best alongside environmental change (school plan + routines + sleep)
- Joined-up support across home/school/services improves outcomes in complex cases

References

Arseneault, L. (2018) 'Annual research review: The persistent and pervasive impact of being bullied in childhood and adolescence: Implications for policy and practice', *Journal of Child Psychology and Psychiatry*, 59(4), pp. 405–421. doi:10.1111/jcpp.12841.

Barron, I.G., Bourgaize, C., Lempertz, D., Swinden, C. and Darker-Smith, S. (2019) 'Eye movement desensitization reprocessing for children and adolescents with post-traumatic stress disorder: A systematic narrative review', *Journal of EMDR Practice and Research*, 13(4), pp. 270–283. doi:10.1891/1933-3196.13.4.270.

Department for Education (DfE) (2024) *Keeping children safe in education: Statutory guidance for schools and colleges*. Available at: www.gov.uk/government/publications/keeping-children-safe-in-education--2 (Accessed: 1 March 2026).

Gee, D.G. and Cohodes, E.M. (2023) 'Leveraging the developmental neuroscience of caregiving to promote resilience among youth exposed to adversity', *Development and Psychopathology*, 35(5), pp. 2168–2185. doi:10.1017/S0954579423001128.

Gunnar, M.R. (2020) 'Early adversity, stress, and neurobehavioral development', *Development and Psychopathology*, 32, pp. 1555–1562. doi:10.1017/S0954579420001649.

Lydecker, J.A. (2022) 'Conceptual application of trauma-focused cognitive behavioral therapy to treat victims of bullying', *Journal of Prevention and Health Promotion*, 3(2), pp. 231–245. doi:10.1177/26320770221074008.

National Institute for Health and Care Excellence (NICE) (2018) *Post-traumatic stress disorder (NG116)*. Available at: www.nice.org.uk/guidance/ng116 (Accessed: 1 March 2026).

National Institute for Health and Care Excellence (NICE) (2019) *Depression in children and young people: Identification and management (NG134)*. Available at: www.nice.org.uk/guidance/ng134 (Accessed: 1 March 2026).

National Institute for Health and Care Excellence (NICE) (2022) *Self-harm: Assessment, management and preventing recurrence (NG225)*. Available at: www.nice.org.uk/guidance/ng225 (Accessed: 1 March 2026).

Sonuga-Barke, E.J.S. (2017) 'Commentary: Extraordinary environments, extreme neuroplasticity and mental disorder – reflections on pathways from adversity to mental disorder prompted by McCrory, Gerin, and Viding (2017)', *Journal of Child Psychology and Psychiatry*, 58(4), pp. 359–360. doi:10.1111/jcpp.12726.

Chapter 5

For Parents

Recognising and Responding to Bullying

Abstract

Parents play a central role in how children recover from bullying. While schools address behaviour, what happens at home strongly influences whether distress becomes entrenched or begins to settle. Research consistently shows that parental warmth, emotional availability and predictable routines reduce the risk of longer-term anxiety, depression and stress-related symptoms following peer victimisation. This chapter explains how parents can respond in ways that reduce shame, strengthen safety and support regulation. It outlines evidence-informed approaches to disclosure, co-regulation, school collaboration and digital safety, and highlights the specific needs of neurodivergent, disabled, and LGBTQ+ children, who experience higher rates of bullying and may face cumulative stress. Practical guidance is provided for supporting recovery, recognising when additional help is needed, and responding constructively if a child has bullied others. The emphasis throughout is on steady protection, emotional connection and coordinated action, grounded in research rather than anecdotal evidence.

This chapter is written for parents and carers who are trying to understand what is happening to their child, and what they can do to help.

In This Chapter:

- What helps most when a child tells you they are being bullied, and what can unintentionally shut them down
- How to recognise signs of bullying when children struggle to put it into words
- How bullying affects emotional wellbeing, behaviour and daily functioning
- Practical ways to support regulation, confidence and recovery at home
- How to work effectively with schools to ensure safety and accountability
- When additional support may be needed, and how to access it

DOI: 10.4324/9781003771777-8

Why Parents Matter in Recovery After Bullying

Bullying does not stop mattering when a child comes home. For many children, the home environment significantly shapes whether distress settles or becomes prolonged.

Longitudinal research has consistently shown that parental warmth and emotional support buffer the mental health impact of peer victimisation. Foundational studies demonstrated that children who experienced high levels of parental support showed fewer later symptoms of anxiety and depression following bullying compared to those who felt unsupported (Bowes et al., 2010; Lereya et al., 2013).

More recent research continues to replicate and extend these findings. Contemporary studies indicate that perceived parental warmth moderates the association between peer victimisation and internalising difficulties, even in adolescence when peer relationships become developmentally central (Fredrick and Demaray, 2018; Kaufman et al., 2020). In other words, supportive parenting remains protective, even as children grow older and peer dynamics intensify (Shaheen et al., 2019).

This buffering effect is not about minimising harm. It reflects the role of caregiving relationships in stress regulation. Developmental neuroscience research shows that supportive caregiving reduces physiological stress reactivity and supports the recovery of emotional regulation systems (Gunnar, 2020; Gee and Cohodes, 2023). Parental warmth does not erase bullying, but reduces the likelihood that distress becomes entrenched.

When children feel believed and protected, the bullying experience is less likely to become internalised as shame or hopelessness (Arseneault, 2018). The same peer event can lead to very different outcomes depending on whether a child feels alone or held within a stable relationship.

Longitudinal evidence supports both the direct and the stress-buffering effects of supportive relationships. In a two-wave study of Australian adolescents, supportive relationships with parents and classmates reduced later psychological distress and decreased the likelihood of persistent bullying victimisation (Healy et al., 2024). Importantly, parental support buffered the impact of bullying on later distress, meaning that victimised adolescents with strong parental relationships showed lower subsequent psychological symptoms than those without such support.

Parent–child and peer relationships influence one another over time. Longitudinal evidence demonstrates bidirectional spillover between parental warmth/rejection and peer victimisation (Kaufman et al., 2020). Higher parental rejection predicts later increases in peer victimisation, and peer victimisation predicts increased parent–child conflict. These cross-domain effects are partly mediated by depressive symptoms. This suggests that strengthening parent–child relationships may reduce risk not only by buffering distress, but by interrupting a potential downward relational spiral.

What to Do First When Your Child Tells You About Bullying

When a child discloses bullying, the initial response shapes whether they continue talking. Many children test disclosure gradually. A dismissive, minimising or panicked response can unintentionally close communication.

Research on parent–child communication shows that validation and a calm presence increase disclosure and reduce shame (Arseneault, 2018). A helpful first response has three components:

1. *Believe and Validate*

- 'Thank you for telling me.'
- 'I'm really glad you told me.'
- 'That shouldn't be happening to you.'

Validation communicates safety. It does not require full details immediately.

2. *Reduce Shame and Self-blame*

Bullying often generates self-blame. Explicitly countering this matters.

- 'This is not your fault.'
- 'You don't deserve to be treated like that.'

Children who internalise blame are at higher risk of anxiety and depression following victimisation (Arseneault, 2018).

3. *Offer Steady Protection*

- 'We will deal with this together.'
- 'You are not on your own.'

Protection should feel calm, not explosive. A highly reactive parental response can increase the child's anxiety about consequences.

If asking questions, keep them gentle and practical:

- 'Where does it usually happen?'
- 'When is it worst?'
- 'Who is there?'

Avoid immediate pressure to confront the bully or 'stand up for yourself' before safety is restored. For some children, particularly those who are younger, neurodivergent or socially vulnerable, this increases risk and reinforces the sense that they must solve the problem alone.

Recognising Bullying When Children Don't Call It Bullying

Many children do not tell a parent directly that they are being bullied. Some feel embarrassed. Some worry it will get worse if adults get involved. Some fear they will be told to 'ignore it', be pushed into confronting someone, or lose access to their phone. Others simply do not have the words yet.

This is why it helps to recognise common signs, not as proof, but as clues that something in your child's world has started to feel unsafe. Patterns matter more than one difficult day.

Common signs at primary age

In younger children, distress often shows up through behaviour and the body rather than through a clear explanation. You might notice:

- More clinginess, tears or meltdowns after school
- Sudden resistance to school, clubs or certain routes
- Stomach aches or headaches that cluster around school mornings
- Sleep changes (nightmares, wanting lights on, waking early)
- Anger that seems out of proportion to the trigger
- Play that becomes more 'mean', fearful or repetitive

If a child cannot explain why, it does not mean nothing is happening. It may mean they are trying to cope without language.

Common signs at secondary age

In older children and teenagers, bullying may be hidden behind withdrawal, irritation or secrecy. You might notice:

- Sharp changes after school (silent, snappy, flat or shut down)
- 'I'm fine' becoming the only answer, paired with avoiding family time
- Friends dropping away, fewer invites, or anxiety about group settings
- Reluctance to participate in Physical Education, lunch or change rooms
- A noticeable dip in concentration, motivation or schoolwork
- Changes in appetite
- Staying up late and struggling to get up, especially on school days

For some teenagers, bullying shows up as anger. For others it shows up as disappearing into their room or going numb. These responses can be mistaken for typical adolescence. The key difference is usually a sustained shift that links to school or peer contact.

Signs that online life may be part of it

Digital harm often leaves distinctive traces. You might see:

- Panic when notifications appear
- Sudden deletion of apps or accounts
- Secrecy about group chats
- 'Doom scrolling' or compulsive checking
- Switching screens quickly when you enter the room
- Being visibly upset after using the phone, but insisting 'it's nothing'

None of these prove cyberbullying. They simply signal: 'something online is not feeling safe'.

How to ask without making it worse

The aim is to open the door, not force a confession. The most helpful questions are calm, specific and non-judgemental:

- 'I've noticed school feels heavier lately. I'm not here to lecture you, I just want to understand.'
- 'Has anyone been making school feel unsafe or stressful?'
- 'Are there any group chats or online stuff that's been upsetting?'

If your child says 'It's fine', keeping the door open matters:

- 'Okay. If you ever want to tell me later, I'm here.'
- 'You won't get in trouble.'

That last sentence is important. Many children stay silent because they fear adult reactions.

If your child only shares small pieces of information

Children often disclose in fragments: one name, one incident, one hint. A steady response helps them continue:

- 'Thank you for telling me that.'
- 'We can go step by step.'
- 'You don't have to carry this alone.'

Your job is not to get every detail in one sitting. Your job is to show your child you can hear difficult things without panicking, blaming or rushing.

Co-regulation: The Science Behind Helping Your Child Calm Down

Children develop self-regulation through repeated experiences of co-regulation with caregivers. This process, widely documented in developmental and attachment research, involves the adult helping the child return to emotional equilibrium during stress. Over time, children internalise these regulatory patterns (Gunnar, 2020; Gee and Cohodes, 2023).

Studies of stress physiology demonstrate that caregiver presence can reduce cortisol responses and improve emotional recovery following social stress (Gunnar, 2020). When parents respond with calm, attuned engagement rather than panic or dismissal, children are more likely to regain cognitive control and problem-solving capacity.

This is particularly relevant after bullying. Peer victimisation activates threat systems associated with vigilance and rumination. Co-regulation interrupts this cycle, allowing the child's nervous system to shift out of defensive mode.

Adolescents also benefit from co-regulation. Although teenagers seek autonomy, parental emotional availability remains strongly associated with reduced internalising symptoms during periods of peer stress (Lereya et al., 2013).

Why Home Routines Support Recovery

Predictable routines play a measurable role in stress regulation. Research on childhood stress indicates that consistent daily rhythms, particularly sleep stability, are associated with more regulated cortisol patterns and improved emotional functioning (Gunnar, 2020).

Bullying often introduces unpredictability and anticipatory anxiety. Structured routines at home counterbalance this instability. Regular sleep, regular meal times and daily check-ins act as environmental signals of safety. While routines alone do not resolve bullying, they create physiological conditions that support recovery.

Sleep disruption is especially significant. Poor sleep amplifies anxiety, emotional reactivity and concentration difficulties. Restoring sleep stability is therefore not a superficial intervention; it is a neurobiological stabiliser.

Supporting Recovery at Home: A Practical Toolkit for the Everyday Moments

Parents often assume that the 'real' work happens at school: reporting, meetings, supervision plans. Those steps are essential. But recovery is often shaped by what happens in the ordinary moments at home, how mornings are handled, what happens after school, how worries are met, and whether the child experiences steady connection without pressure.

This section is not about perfect parenting. It is about the small, repeatable practices that help children feel safer and more settled over time.

1) *The School-morning Problem: Keeping It Predictable without Forcing It*

For many children, mornings are the hardest point of the day. Even when bullying has reduced, the body can still expect threat. Parents often find themselves caught between two fears: pushing too hard and breaking trust, or accommodating so much that school becomes impossible.

A middle path is *predictable structure plus emotional calm*.

Helpful principles:

- Keep mornings *short and simple*: fewer questions, fewer negotiations.
- Use *small, neutral prompts* rather than big pep talks.
- Separate emotion from action: you can validate feelings while still moving forward.

Useful phrases:

- 'I can see this feels hard. We'll take it step by step.'
- 'You don't have to feel brave to go. You just have to go with support.'
- 'We have a plan for today. You know who to go to if it feels unsafe.'

If your child becomes distressed, it can help to use a 'two-minute settle' before leaving:

- A drink of water
- Slow breathing for 30 seconds
- A short grounding routine (feet on the floor, naming five things you can see)
- A clear reminder of the first safe adult they'll see

The aim is not to eliminate fear. It is to prevent fear from taking over the whole day.

2) *After-school Decompression: Why It Matters*

Many children hold themselves together at school and unravel at home. This can look like tears, anger, exhaustion or complete withdrawal.

Parents sometimes interpret this as 'school must be fine, they coped all day'. Often it means the opposite: your child has used all their energy to survive socially.

A helpful routine is a protected decompression window:

- A period of 20–40 minutes with low demands
- Food and drink available
- Minimal questioning
- A predictable activity (shower, snack, favourite programme, quiet time, walking the dog)

A simple sentence can help:

- 'You don't have to talk yet. Let your body land first.'

3) Daily Check-ins that Don't Feel like Interrogation

Parents understandably want details. Children often don't. The goal is to keep the conversation open without making every evening feel like an interview.

Options that work well:

- **Best/hard/help**
  'Best moment today?'
  'Hardest moment?'
  'What do you need from me tonight?'
- **Traffic lights**
  'Green, amber or red day?'
  (If red: 'What was the hardest part?' If green: 'What helped?')
- **One number**
  'If 0 is "calm" and 10 is "overwhelmed", what number are you now?'

For younger children, indirect check-ins can be easier:

- Drawing a 'school day weather report' (sunny/cloudy/stormy)
- Using toys to show where they felt safe or unsafe
- Asking about 'the kindest person' and 'the hardest moment' rather than 'who bullied you?'.

4) When your Child Replays Events Over and Over

After bullying, some children replay scenes in their mind, especially at night. Parents may hear the same story repeatedly or see the child getting stuck on 'why me?'. This can be distressing to witness.

A parent-safe approach is:

1. **Name it without judgement**
   'Your mind keeps going back to it.'
2. **Validate the reason**
   'That makes sense, your brain is trying to work out how to stay safe.'
3. **Gently shift to the present**
   'Let's bring you back to now. What helps your body settle?'
4. **Offer a container**
   'We can talk about it for five minutes, then we'll do something that helps your body feel calmer.'

This avoids dismissing the child while also stopping rumination becoming the whole evening.

5) Confidence-building Through Competence (Not Popularity)

Bullying often attacks identity. Children can start to believe they are 'less than', weak, or unwanted. One of the most protective things parents can do is help the child experience competence again, in any domain.

Choose activities where:

- Success is likely
- Adult support is kind and predictable
- There is structure (clear rules, shared tasks)

Examples:

- Walking, swimming, dance, martial arts with a supportive instructor
- Music, art, coding, drama
- Volunteering, community groups, youth clubs
- A meaningful role at home (cooking one meal a week, caring for a pet, organising something)

These experiences quietly rebuild: 'I can do things. I belong somewhere.'

6) Handling the Urge to 'Fix' It Quickly

Parents often feel pressure to act immediately, contact multiple staff, or repeatedly ask for updates. Some action is necessary, but too much intensity can increase a child's fear ('this must be really dangerous') or communicate panic. A useful rule is: be active behind the scenes, and calm in front of your child.

- Do the emails, meetings and documentation in adult space.
- Give your child short, reassuring updates:

'I spoke to the school. Here's the plan for tomorrow.'

7) *Repair After a Difficult Conversation*

Even supportive parents sometimes snap, especially when tired or frightened. Repair is powerful.

Repair sounds like:

- 'I'm sorry I got sharp. I was worried, not angry with you.'
- 'Let's try again. I want to listen properly.'
- 'You didn't do anything wrong by telling me.'

Children learn safety not from perfect conversations, but from knowing you return and repair.

A Parent Action Plan (First 48 Hours, First Week, Weeks 2–6)

A simple parent action plan: the first 48 hours, the first week, and the next month

Parents often feel pressure to fix bullying quickly. That urgency makes sense, but the most effective approach is usually two-stranded: *calm emotional support* (so your child feels safe enough to talk) and *practical protection* (so harm reduces and safety becomes real).

First 48 hours: calm, contain and gather the basics

In the first day or two, your child may still be running on adrenaline. Even if they look 'fine', their body can be in alert mode. In this early window, 'calm first, then plan' matters more than the perfect words.

What helps most:

- Keep your voice steady and your sentences short.
- Validate: 'That shouldn't be happening.'
- Reduce shame: 'This is not your fault.'
- Protect: 'We'll deal with it together.'

Then gather only what you need:

- What happens most often?
- Where and when is it worst?

- Who is involved or present?
- Is anything happening online too?

If your child becomes overwhelmed, pause:

- 'We don't have to go through it all tonight. I believe you. We'll take it step by step.'

This is often more effective than a long interrogation, which can make children shut down.

First week: visible safety and a plan your child can rely on
In week one, the goals are: reduce exposure to harm, stop escalation, and make safety predictable.

Helpful steps include:

1. *Contact the school* and ask what will happen next, and by when.
2. *Ask for a named adult* your child can go to immediately.
3. *Ask about high-risk times* (arrival, corridors, lunch, dismissal) and what supervision/support will be in place.
4. *Keep routines steady at home,* especially sleep and meals.
5. *Avoid pressuring your child to confront peers* before adults have put safety in place.

If bullying is also online, begin calm evidence capture and reporting (see Cyberbullying section below), but avoid a sudden phone ban unless there is immediate risk. Many young people stop disclosing if they fear losing their phone, because it feels like they are losing their social world.

Weeks 2–6: rebuilding confidence and belonging
A common parent experience is: 'The bullying has stopped, but my child still isn't okay.' That lag is normal. Recovery is often a slow return of everyday signs: better sleep, fewer body complaints, less dread, more humour, more willingness to engage.

What helps in this phase:

- *One stable belonging point* each week (club, hobby, group, responsibility). Belonging doesn't have to be popularity. It has to be reliable.
- *Confidence through competence* (something your child can succeed at: movement, music, art, coding, volunteering, a role at home).
- *Short daily check-ins,* not long interrogations. A simple pattern is:
    - 'Best moment today?'

  - 'Hardest moment?'
  - 'What do you need from me tonight?'
- *Plan for setbacks.* Setbacks often happen around transitions, exams, renewed peer contact or online triggers. A calm response is an early response: restore routines, reinforce school safety steps and return to basics (sleep, food, movement, predictable check-ins).

If you remember one thing: *recovery is built through repeated experiences of safety,* not through one big conversation.

Working with Schools Effectively

Most parents do not want conflict with the school. They want safety. The challenge is that school responses vary, and vague reassurance can unintentionally leave children feeling alone. A calm, specific, persistent approach is usually the most effective.

What to ask for in the first contact

Aim for clear answers to four questions:

1. Who is the lead person managing this?
2. What immediate steps are being taken this week to reduce harm?
3. What should my child do tomorrow if something happens again?
4. When will we review progress?

A helpful line that keeps the tone practical:

- 'My priority is that my child feels safe enough to attend and learn. What are the concrete steps being taken this week?'

Ask about high-risk times (where plans often fail)

Bullying often happens in predictable places and times: corridors, lunch, toilets, change rooms, arrival/dismissal and online spillover. Ask directly:

- 'What supervision plan is in place during the times this tends to happen?'
- 'How will my child access help quickly if they feel unsafe?'

A named adult matters

'Telling a teacher' is too vague for many children. Ask:

- 'Who is the named person my child goes to first?'
- 'Where will that person be at lunch?'
- 'What happens if that person is absent?'

Predictability reduces fear.

Why written follow-up helps
After a call or meeting, it is reasonable to email a brief summary:

- What was agreed
- Who will do what
- When it will be reviewed

This is not about being difficult. It prevents drift and misunderstandings.

If the school's response is vague
If you hear, 'We'll keep an eye on it', calmly ask:

- 'What does that look like day to day?'
- 'Who is responsible for that supervision?'
- 'How will we know whether it's improving?'

You are asking for clarity, not demanding punishment.

If bullying involves online spaces
If peers are from school, ask how the school will respond. Online harm can still affect attendance, wellbeing and peer relationships. You can say:

- 'This is online, but it's affecting school life and wellbeing. What safeguarding steps will be taken?'

When you may need to escalate
If harm continues, escalate through the school's formal pathways. Keep communication factual: dates, patterns and impact (sleep, attendance, fear, withdrawal). Consistency matters more than intensity: calm messages, written follow-up and clear review dates.

A short sample email (copy and paste)
Subject: Safety and support plan for [Child's name]

Dear [Name/Year Head/Safeguarding Lead],

[Child's name] has told me they are experiencing bullying. I am concerned about their wellbeing and would like to understand what immediate steps will be taken to ensure their safety.

Could you please confirm:

- Who the named staff contact will be for [Child's name] if they feel unsafe
- What supervision/support will be in place during the times/locations where this tends to occur

- How incidents/actions will be recorded and communicated
- When we can review progress (a date/time would be helpful)

My priority is that [Child's name] feels safe enough to attend and learn. Thank you for your help.

Kind regards,
[Your name]

Supporting Neurodivergent, Disabled and LGBTQ+ Children

Children who are neurodivergent, disabled or LGBTQ+ experience elevated rates of bullying across multiple studies. While earlier research established this pattern, more recent meta-analyses and population studies confirm that these disparities remain significant (Johns et al., 2020).

Importantly, newer research has strengthened the understanding of protective mechanisms. Family affirmation and acceptance are associated with significantly lower rates of depression, self-harm and suicidality among LGBTQ+ adolescents. Similarly, parental advocacy and explicit validation improve resilience outcomes in neurodivergent youth facing peer victimisation (Park et al., 2020).

These findings suggest that identity-affirming parenting is not a political stance; it is a measurable protective factor.

Recent evidence further clarifies the mechanisms through which family and school environments buffer suicide risk among LGBTQ+ youth. A 2024 scoping review synthesising 66 studies found that protective factors operate across ecological levels, with family connectedness, supportive adults, at-school safety and inclusive policies consistently associated with reduced suicidality (Wallace et al., 2024). Similarly, a 2025 scoping review of school-based suicide prevention efforts concluded that LGBTQ+-affirming environments, inclusive anti-bullying policies and visible adult allies reduce suicidal thoughts and behaviours among LGBTQ+ youth (Stilwell et al., 2026).

These findings reinforce that parental affirmation and advocacy are not optional extras; they are measurable protective factors.

Recent research confirms significantly elevated bullying rates among autistic pre-adolescents. In a 2024 study of Spanish schoolchildren, 58 percent of autistic participants reported bullying victimisation, representing a three-fold increase in risk compared to neurotypical peers (Morales-Hidalgo et al., 2024). Victimisation was associated with greater restrictive behaviours and increased emotional difficulties. These findings reinforce the need for proactive advocacy and structured protection for neurodivergent children in mainstream settings.

Parental Affirmation is Protective

Family acceptance is one of the strongest protective factors against mental health difficulties in LGBTQ+ youth. Even small signals of acceptance, using a chosen name, challenging prejudice and expressing pride can reduce the risk of depression and suicidality.

For neurodivergent children, explicitly valuing difference reduces shame and supports resilience.

Avoid messages implying that safety depends on conformity. Statements such as 'try to fit in more' may unintentionally increase self-blame.

Advocacy Matters

Identity-based bullying requires a systemic response. Schools must address discriminatory behaviour explicitly. Parental advocacy is often necessary to ensure safeguarding is proportionate and consistent (Department for Education, 2024).

Recognise Cumulative Stress

Bullying may intersect with discrimination, sensory overload or exclusion (Lee et al., 2025). Cumulative stress can intensify distress and delay recovery (Gunnar, 2020).

Support may therefore need to be more protective and sustained.

Identity-based Examples for Parents

Practical Examples: What Support Looks Like at Home (And What to Ask of the School)

The evidence is clear that risk is unevenly distributed: neurodivergent, disabled and LGBTQ+ children experience higher rates of bullying, and identity-based bullying can carry an added layer of shame and fear (Morales-Hidalgo et al., 2024; Wallace et al., 2024; Stilwell et al., 2026). What parents often need in this situation is not more theory, but clear examples of what helps in real life.

The examples below are not 'scripts to memorise'. They are illustrations of the kind of steady, protective responses that keep a child talking and reduce shame.

Example 1: An autistic child who is being targeted for being 'different'

A parent might notice their child becoming more rigid, exhausted or distressed after school, or refusing certain lessons or social times. Sometimes the bullying is overt; sometimes it is repetitive teasing, exclusion, mimicry or 'baiting' designed to provoke a reaction.

What helps at home

- Name the pattern without blaming your child:
  'It sounds like they're choosing to target you because they notice what's different. That is not your fault.'
- Offer a clear protection message:
  'My job is to help make this safer. You don't have to handle it alone.'
- Reduce the 'fix yourself' pressure:
  Avoid: 'Try to act more normal/fit in.'
  Prefer: 'You shouldn't have to change who you are to be safe.'
- Make the plan concrete:
  'If it happens at break, what's the quickest safe step? Who do you go to first?'
  (Neurodivergent children often do best with clarity rather than broad reassurance.)

What to ask of school

- A named safe adult and a predictable place your child can go.
- Supervision for the settings where the pattern occurs (often break/lunch/transition times).
- A plan that recognises that repeated 'low-level' targeting can have a high impact over time.
- Staff awareness that a distressed reaction may be the result of provocation, not 'behaviour for no reason'.

Recent evidence highlights the high prevalence of victimisation among autistic pre-adolescents and the links with increased emotional difficulties, underlining why proactive protection matters (Morales-Hidalgo et al., 2024).

Example 2: A disabled child being bullied about appearance, mobility or support needs

Bullying can include staring, comments, exclusion ('we don't want you in our team'), taking photos, mocking aids or social media posts. Even when the incidents look 'small' to adults, the cumulative message can be: 'You don't belong.'

What helps at home

- Affirm dignity clearly:
  'Your body/support needs are not the problem. Their behaviour is the problem.'

- Protect against internalised shame:
  'If people are cruel about disability, it says something about prejudice, not about your worth.'
- Keep routines steady during stressful periods:
  Predictability matters when the outside world feels unsafe (Gunnar, 2020).
- Give recovery somewhere else to live:
  Support one area where your child feels competent and valued (hobby, role, interest group), so confidence is not entirely dependent on peer approval.

What to ask of the school

- A clear anti-discrimination response (not only 'friendship issues' language).
- The monitoring of high-risk locations (e.g. toilets, corridors, playground edges).
- Action on image-based behaviour if photos are involved.
- A plan for safe participation (so 'protecting' does not become isolating).

Example 3: An LGBTQ+ young person who is being targeted online and at school

For some young people, bullying is directly tied to identity. This can include slurs, rumours, threats of being outed or harassment in group chats. The fear is not only about harm, it can be about exposure and loss of control.

Recent reviews emphasise that protective factors operate across systems: family connectedness, supportive adults and visibly inclusive environments reduce risk, including risk related to suicidality (Wallace et al., 2024; Stilwell et al., 2026). Parents often matter most because they can reduce shame and increase safety at the same time.

What helps at home

- Make acceptance explicit, not assumed:
  'I love you exactly as you are. You don't have to hide from me.'
  'You deserve safety and respect.'
- Use the language your child asks for:
  Names and pronouns are not a debate at home, they are a signal of safety.
- Avoid accidental minimising:
  Avoid: 'Ignore it, they're just being stupid.'
  Prefer: 'What they're doing is wrong, and we'll work out the safest response together.'
- Maintain dignity when taking action:
  'I won't rush to do things behind your back, but I also won't leave you unprotected. Let's plan the next step together.'

What to ask of the school

- A clear statement of what the school will do to address discriminatory bullying (not only general behaviour messaging).
- Visible adult allies and safe reporting routes.
- A plan that recognises the overlap between online harm and in-school dynamics (Department for Education, 2024).

A final practical principle for identity-based bullying

When bullying targets identity, children often need *more protection, not more pressure to change*. The most helpful parent stance is usually: calm acceptance at home, clear advocacy with the school, and steady routines that help the stress system settle over time (Gunnar, 2020; Department for Education, 2024).

Cyberbullying: What Parents Need to Know

Cyberbullying can feel frightening because it follows children into their homes. Unlike face-to-face bullying, it can happen at any hour, spread quickly and feel hard to escape. Research links cyberbullying with increased anxiety, low mood, sleep disruption and school avoidance, particularly when it happens alongside in-person bullying.

A parent's goal is usually twofold: *reduce harm and keep your child talking*. If a child fears losing their phone or being blamed, they may stop disclosing. This is why a calm, collaborative approach is usually more effective than sudden bans.

A practical framework that helps

1. Keep communication open
   Ask about online life in a curious, non-judgemental way:
   - 'Any group chats feeling stressful?'
   - 'Anything online making school harder?'
   - 'Has anything been shared that upset you?'

   If your child is reluctant:
   - 'You don't have to show me everything. I just want to help you feel safer.'
2. Capture evidence calmly
   If there are harmful messages or images, screenshots can help with reporting and school action. Try not to turn home into an 'investigation centre'. A simple approach is:
   - 'Let's save what matters, then we'll stop looking at it for tonight.'

3. Block and report
   Use platform tools to block and report. If the people involved are from school, involve school leadership, because online harm often affects school life and wellbeing.
4. Make a digital safety agreement together
   Collaborative boundaries are more likely to be followed than sudden punishments. Agree:
   - Which apps are used
   - When devices are off (especially before sleep)
   - What your child will do if something upsetting appears
   - Who they will tell first
5. Watch for threat-checking spirals
   Some young people repeatedly check their phone because they are monitoring danger. It can look like 'they won't put it down', but it is often fear-driven. If you notice compulsive checking, respond with support rather than criticism:
   - 'It looks hard to switch off. Let's put the phone in the kitchen for 20 minutes and do something together.'

A strong, secure parent–child relationship can reduce the psychological impact of cyberbullying even when exposure cannot be fully prevented, which is another reason to prioritise calm presence and continued conversation.

Cyberbullying Scripts, Decision Tree and a Digital Safety Agreement

Cyberbullying can be hard for parents because it often arrives with uncertainty: you may not know what was said, who has seen it, or whether it will escalate. Children may also resist showing messages, either because they feel ashamed or because they fear losing their phone.

Research indicates that the impact of cyberbullying is shaped not only by the online event itself, but by whether young people feel supported and safe enough to disclose (Zhu et al., 2021). The aim is to reduce harm while keeping communication open.

If your child won't show you messages

A common mistake is escalating pressure: 'Show me right now.' That can push disclosure further away. A calmer approach is to offer choices and control:

- 'You don't have to show me everything. I believe you.'
- 'Would it help if you just told me the general type of thing, messages, images, threats, rumours?'
- 'Would you rather show me one screenshot, or tell me the worst part in words?'
- 'My job is to help you feel safer, not to take everything away.'

If your child is worried about losing their phone, you can say explicitly:

- 'I'm not going to punish you for telling me. Let's work out a plan together.'

A simple decision guide (parents often find this clarifying)

Step 1: Is there immediate risk or serious coercion?
Examples include threats, blackmail, pressure to share images or fear of physical harm.

If yes: prioritise safety and follow your school's safeguarding route and local guidance (Department for Education, 2024). If you are worried about immediate safety, seek urgent professional support.

Step 2: Is it ongoing and spreading, or is it contained?

- *Contained* (one person; limited platform): block/report and protect sleep.
- *Spreading* (group chat, reposting, multiple accounts): evidence capture + school involvement is usually needed because peer dynamics often continue in person.

Step 3: Is the school involved (same peers)?
If the people involved are from school, online harm usually affects school wellbeing and attendance. It is reasonable to involve the school leadership and request a clear plan (Department for Education, 2024).

What to screenshot (without turning home into a 'case file')

Evidence capture is useful, but it can also keep children stuck staring at harmful content. Aim for 'enough, then stop'.

- Capture: usernames, dates/times, the core harmful messages/images and any threats.
- Then say: 'We've saved what we need. We're closing it for tonight.'

Scripts for common situations

If your child blames themselves:

- 'Nothing you did makes it okay for someone to target you.'

If your child feels embarrassed:

- 'I'm not disappointed in you. I'm concerned about what was done to you.'

If your child says, 'don't tell the school':

- 'I hear you. We'll go carefully. My job is to protect you, we can plan what to share and who to speak to first.'

If your child is panic-checking constantly:

- 'It makes sense you're checking; your brain is trying to stop surprises.'
- 'Let's take a 20-minute break from the phone and do something that helps your body settle.'

(Repeated checking can be threat-monitoring; responding with calm support helps more than criticism. Stronger parent–child connection can buffer impact even when exposure can't be fully prevented (Zhu et al., 2021).)

A simple digital safety agreement (copy and adapt)

This is not about control. It's about predictability and support.

Our digital safety agreement

- Apps we use: ____________________________
- Apps we are pausing/limiting for now: ___________________________
- Device-free bedtime begins at: ___________________
- If something upsetting appears, the first step is:
  ☐ don't reply ☐ screenshot ☐ block ☐ tell a trusted adult
- The first adult I will tell is: ____________________________
- If I don't want to talk, I can send a signal (emoji/text word): ________
- If things escalate (threats/blackmail), we will: ______________________

Involving school: a parent-safe line

- 'This is happening online, but it's affecting wellbeing and school life. What safeguarding steps will be taken and when will we review progress?' (Department for Education, 2024)

Protecting sleep (often the quickest win)

Cyberbullying often disrupts sleep. Sleep stabilisation is one of the strongest 'first recovery wins' because it improves emotional control the next day. Consider:

- Device-free time before bed
- Charging phones outside bedrooms where possible (agreed, not imposed)
- Calming routines that are consistent (Gunnar, 2020)

Friendship Repair and Confidence Rebuilding

Helping your child rebuild confidence and friendships
Bullying is social harm. It doesn't only create fear, it often damages trust and belonging. Parents often focus on stopping the bullying (which is essential), but children also need help rebuilding their sense of safety in groups afterwards.

Rebuild in small, structured steps

1. Start with one safer connection
   Instead of pushing your child into big friendship groups, support one safer person:
   - A cousin, neighbour or family friend
   - One consistently kind peer
   - A small club environment where attention is on an interest, not popularity
2. Choose belonging that is not status-based
   Belonging is easier to rebuild in settings with shared structure: art, drama, coding, music, youth groups, volunteering, sport with a supportive coach. These settings reduce the pressure of 'finding your place!
3. Support gentle social practice
   Some children benefit from rehearsing short lines so they don't freeze:
   - 'No thanks!'
   - 'Please stop!'
   - 'I'm going to sit here!'
   - 'I'm going to get a teacher!'

This is not about blaming the child to 'handle it better'. It's about giving them words so they feel less powerless.

4. Notice shame and challenge it gently
   Bullying often leaves behind shame thoughts: 'It's me', 'I'm embarrassing', 'Everyone hates me'. You don't need therapy language to respond:
   - 'It makes sense you feel that way after what happened.'
   - 'Being targeted doesn't mean you deserved it.'
   - 'This says something about their behaviour, not your worth.'
5. Give recovery somewhere else to live
   If school is the main arena of harm, help your child build at least one area of life that is separate: a hobby, role or group outside school. It gives the nervous system a break and restores identity beyond 'the bullied child'.

When to Seek Extra Help: Guidance for Parents

Most children show some gradual improvement once bullying stops and adults respond consistently. However, there are times when extra support is needed. Seeking help is not a sign you have failed. It is a sensible response when distress is lasting, escalating or getting in the way of daily life.

A helpful way to think about this is in three bands: ongoing distress, significant impact and urgent risk. The examples below are not a checklist for diagnosis. They are signposts that it may be time to involve a general practitioner (GP), school mental health lead or specialist services, depending on what is available locally (National Institute for Health and Care Excellence, 2018; National Institute for Health and Care Excellence, 2019; National Institute for Health and Care Excellence, 2022; Department for Education, 2024).

1) Ongoing Distress: When It Is Not Settling

Consider speaking with school support or your GP if your child:

- Remains consistently upset, fearful or withdrawn for more than a few weeks
- Is increasingly irritable or tearful at home
- Seems 'on edge' most of the time, even when nothing obvious has happened that day
- Avoids things they previously enjoyed, including friends or hobbies
- Has sleep disruption that continues (difficulty falling asleep, nightmares, waking early)

Many children will have some of these signs briefly. What matters is persistence, and whether your child seems to be getting 'stuck' rather than slowly improving.

2) *Significant Impact: When Daily Life Starts Shrinking*

Additional support is often appropriate when bullying has begun to affect functioning.
This might include:

- *School avoidance* that persists (not just the occasional difficult morning)
- Regular physical complaints on school days (stomach aches, headaches, nausea)
- A noticeable drop in concentration, confidence or participation in learning
- A marked change in eating or appetite that does not settle
- Repeated 'replaying' of upsetting moments, or strong distress when reminded of school or peers
- Becoming socially isolated, with friendships falling away or fear of group settings

If your child is missing significant school, the most helpful response is usually coordinated: home, school and health professionals working together. Waiting can sometimes make return harder, because avoidance becomes more entrenched.

3) *Urgent Risk: When to Seek Help Immediately*

If your child talks about wanting to die, mentions self-harm, appears at immediate risk or you are seriously concerned about their safety, seek urgent professional help immediately. This may be through your GP, local crisis services, NHS 111/999 depending on your situation, or your setting's safeguarding lead. National Institute for Health and Care Excellence (NICE) guidance is clear that self-harm and suicidality require timely assessment and support (National Institute for Health and Care Excellence, 2022).

Signs that require urgent action include:

- Your child talking about not wanting to be here, feeling hopeless or wanting to disappear
- Self-harm or evidence you suspect self-harm
- Sudden escalation in risk-taking behaviour
- Threats, coercion or exploitation linked to bullying (including image-based abuse or blackmail) (Department for Education, 2024)

You do not need to wait for certainty. If you are worried, act.

What Tends to Help

You do not need to pick the 'perfect' support first time. Effective help is usually a combination of:

- *Practical protection* (bullying stopped, risk managed, clear safety plans)
- *Relational support* (a trusted adult connection, steady home routines)
- *Skills support* (help with managing worry, shame, re-engagement, confidence)

Where structured talking support is recommended, approaches commonly include CBT-based support for anxiety/low mood, family-based support for routines and communication, and trauma-informed approaches where children are experiencing persistent fear responses or unwanted replays of events (National Institute for Health and Care Excellence, 2018; National Institute for Health and Care Excellence, 2019).

If Your Child has Bullied Someone Else

Discovering your child has harmed another child can feel upsetting, embarrassing or frightening. It may also bring up fear: 'What does this say about my child?' The goal is accountability without shame-labelling. Children need clear boundaries and clear values, but they do not benefit from being defined by their worst behaviour.

Bullying behaviour can have many drivers: copying what they have seen, trying to gain status, struggling with impulse control, reacting to insecurity, or managing stress badly. None of these excuses harm, but understanding the driver helps you respond effectively.

A Steady Approach that Works

1) Stay calm and gather facts

Try to avoid reacting with humiliation or panic. Ask:

- 'Tell me what happened.'
- 'What was going on for you in that moment?'
- 'Who else was there?'
- 'Has this happened before?'

If your child minimises ('It was a joke'), keep your response steady:

- 'If it hurt someone or made them feel unsafe, it's not a joke. We need to take this seriously.'

2) Make expectations clear: harm must stop
Children need clarity:

- 'This stops now!'
- 'In our family we do not use power to frighten or humiliate others.'

Be direct about behaviour, not identity:

- Avoid: 'You're a bully!'
- Prefer: 'That was bullying behaviour. It caused harm.'

3) Focus on empathy and impact
Ask questions that build perspective:

- 'How do you think it felt for them?'
- 'What might they be thinking about school tomorrow?'
- 'If it happened to you, what would you want adults to do?'

4) Agree on consequences that teach responsibility
Consequences should be linked to learning and repair, not humiliation. Examples:

- Loss of a privilege linked to the behaviour (e.g. group chat access if that was used to harm)
- Writing a reflection (not posted publicly)
- Supervised use of online spaces
- Structured apology only when safe and appropriate (and not forced)

5) Involve the school and work with them
If patterns persist, school involvement is important. Ask:

- What the school response plan is
- What supervision and boundaries will be in place
- What support is being offered (social skills, mentoring, pastoral support)

6) Look for underlying needs
If bullying behaviour is repeated, consider whether there are unmet needs such as:

- Friendship insecurity
- Difficulty managing anger
- Impulsivity
- Distress at home or at school
- Social misunderstanding (particularly for some neurodivergent children)

The solution is rarely 'more punishment'. It is usually clear boundaries plus support.

Parent Wellbeing: Staying Steady without Carrying It Alone

Supporting your child without burning out

When your child is being bullied, it can trigger intense protective instincts: anger, fear, guilt and a constant urge to act. These reactions are normal. They are also exhausting.

Steadiness doesn't mean doing it all alone. It means getting support so you can keep showing up calmly.

Common parent traps

- *Over-questioning:* understandable, but can feel like pressure to a child. A short daily check-in often works better.
- *Escalating in front of your child:* adult anger can increase a child's sense that everything is dangerous. Keep adult problem-solving conversations adult-only.
- *Treating recovery like a deadline:* recovery is often gradual. Slow progress is a cue to strengthen support, not withdraw it.

A protective pattern for parents

- One trusted person you can talk to (friend, family member, school lead, GP)
- One small daily reset (walk, shower, time outside)
- One planned moment of connection with your child that is not 'about bullying' (meal, show, game, walk)

Children recover best when at least one adult remains emotionally available and consistent over time. You do not have to do that perfectly, you just have to keep showing up.

Common Parent Dilemmas

Parents often face the same sticking points, even when they are doing many things well. The aim in each situation is the same: keep your child talking, reduce exposure to harm, and make adult protection predictable.

'My Child Begged Me Not to Tell the School.'

This is extremely common. Children often fear escalation, embarrassment or being seen as 'snitching'. Start by acknowledging the fear, then offer a planned approach rather than a sudden action.

Helpful responses include:

- 'I hear you. I won't rush into anything without telling you what I'm doing.'
- 'But I also can't leave you unprotected. Let's plan the safest next step together.'
- 'We can start small, a quiet conversation with one named person, and review.'

If your child agrees, involve them in choices: who to speak to first, what to share, and how to protect privacy. If risk is high (threats, coercion, serious harm), you may need to act even without consent. In that case, keep your child informed and supported as you follow safeguarding routes (Department for Education, 2024; National Institute for Health and Care Excellence, 2022).

'The School Says there's "No Evidence".'

Bullying isn't always a single dramatic incident. It can be repeated exclusion, subtle intimidation and patterns that are hard to capture in one moment. If the school response is 'no evidence', shift the conversation towards pattern and impact.

You can say:

- 'I understand this may not be visible in one incident. I'm concerned about a pattern and the impact on wellbeing and attendance.'
- 'What steps will be taken to monitor high-risk times and settings for the next two weeks?'
- 'When can we review what has been observed?'

Keep a brief record at home: dates, what your child reports, changes in sleep/attendance and what actions have been taken. This isn't about building a case; it's about making adult responses consistent and reviewable.

'The Other Child is "Struggling Too", and the School Wants Us to be Understanding.'

Two things can be true: another child may be struggling, and your child still deserves safety. Support for the other child should never come at the cost of leaving your child exposed.

A calm line that holds boundaries is:

- 'I can understand there may be wider needs. My priority is that my child is safe and able to learn. What safeguards are in place to prevent further harm?'

You can be compassionate without accepting ongoing risk.

'My Child has Become Angry or Aggressive at Home.'

After bullying, some children live in a state of tension and react strongly to small frustrations. This can be frightening for parents, especially if it's new behaviour. Try to treat it as a stress signal first, while still holding clear boundaries.

What often helps:

- Keep limits simple: 'I won't let you hurt anyone or break things.'
- Reduce lectures in the moment. Calm first, talk later.
- After the storm: 'That was a big reaction. I wonder if your body is still carrying a lot from school.'

If anger is escalating, or your child is becoming unsafe, it's appropriate to seek additional support through school, your GP or local services (National Institute for Health and Care Excellence, 2019).

'My Child is Checking their Phone Constantly, but They Won't Show Me What's Happening.'

Compulsive checking is often threat-monitoring, trying to prevent surprises. If you respond with criticism or confiscation, disclosure can reduce. Aim for collaborative structure.

Try:

- 'It looks hard to switch off. Let's take a 20-minute break together.'
- 'Would you rather tell me the type of thing, without showing me?'

Then agree on a small boundary that supports sleep (for example, charging devices outside bedrooms) as a joint plan rather than a punishment (Gunnar, 2020).

'The Bullying has Stopped, but My Child Still Isn't Okay.'

This is one of the most common and most confusing experiences for parents. A child's body can stay on alert even when the immediate threat has reduced.

The aim now is not just 'stopping bullying', but *restoring safety through repetition:* predictable routines, steady check-ins and rebuilding belonging in small steps (Gunnar, 2020; Gee and Cohodes, 2023).

If distress remains high, daily life keeps shrinking (sleep, school attendance, isolation), or your child expresses hopelessness or self-harm, seek additional support and follow local guidance (National Institute for Health and Care Excellence, 2018; National Institute for Health and Care Excellence, 2019; National Institute for Health and Care Excellence, 2022).

Key Messages for Parents

Recovery is shaped by safety, connection and consistency.
Calm first, then problem-solve.
Parental warmth is protective.
Routines regulate stress systems.
Some children require more advocacy because of identity-based vulnerability.
Cyberbullying requires collaborative digital safety and school involvement.
Additional support is appropriate when distress persists or escalates.

Key Takeaways

- Believe first. Kids disclose when they feel safe, not interrogated.
- Regulate before you problem-solve: calm voice, steady presence, predictable routine.
- Keep brief notes (dates, what happened, who you spoke to) so the school's action stays clear.
- If bullying targets identity, the priority is *affirmation at home + firm advocacy at school,* not asking the child to 'change themselves'.
- Cyberbullying: keep communication open, screenshot *enough,* block/report, protect sleep, and agree on a simple digital safety plan together.
- Escalate for extra help if you see school refusal, panic, persistent sleep disruption, self-harm thoughts or rapid deterioration.
- If your child has bullied others: hold boundaries, understand what's driving it, and focus on repair + safer skills.

References

Arseneault, L. (2018) 'Annual research review: The persistent and pervasive impact of being bullied in childhood and adolescence: Implications for policy and practice', *Journal of Child Psychology and Psychiatry,* 59(4), pp. 405–421. doi:10.1111/jcpp.12841.

Bowes, L., Maughan, B., Caspi, A., Moffitt, T.E. and Arseneault, L. (2010) 'Families promote emotional and behavioural resilience to bullying: Evidence of an environmental effect', *Journal of Child Psychology and Psychiatry,* 51(7), pp. 809–817. doi:10.1111/j.1469-7610.2010.02216.x.

Department for Education (DfE) (2024) *Keeping children safe in education: Statutory guidance for schools and colleges*. Available at: www.gov.uk/government/publications/keeping-children-safe-in-education--2 (Accessed: 1 March 2026).

Fredrick, S.S. and Demaray, M.K. (2018) 'Peer victimization and suicidal ideation: The role of gender depression in a school-based sample', *Journal of School Psychology*, 67, pp. 1–15. doi:10. 1016/j.jsp.2018.02.001.

Gee, D.G. and Cohodes, E.M. (2023) 'Leveraging the developmental neuroscience of caregiving to promote resilience among youth exposed to adversity', *Development and Psychopathology*, 35(5), pp. 2168–2185. doi:10.1017/S0954579423001128.

Gunnar, M.R. (2020) 'Early adversity, stress, and neurobehavioral development', *Development and Psychopathology*, 32, pp. 1555–1562. doi:10.1017/S0954579420001649.

Healy, K.L., Scott, J.G. and Thomas, H.J. (2024) 'The protective role of supportive relationships in mitigating bullying victimization and psychological distress in adolescents', *Journal of Child and Family Studies*, 33, pp. 3211–3228. doi:10.1007/s10826-024-02891-2.

Johns, M.M., Lowry, R., Haderxhanaj, L.T., Rasberry, C.N., Robin, L., Scales, L., Stone, D. and Suarez, N.A. (2020) 'Trends in violence victimization and suicide risk by sexual identity among high school students—Youth Risk Behavior Survey, United States, 2015–2019', *MMWR Supplements*, 69(Suppl-1), pp. 19–27. doi:10.15585/mmwr.su6901a3.

Kaufman, T.M.L., Kretschmer, T., Huitsing, G. and Veenstra, R. (2020) 'Caught in a vicious cycle? Explaining bidirectional spillover between parent-child relationships and peer victimization', *Development and Psychopathology*, 32, pp. 11–20. doi:10.1017/S0954579418001360.

Lee, K.H., Park, M., Shin, J., Lee, J., Yoo, J.H., Chun, J. and Kim, J.-W. (2025) 'The moderating role of hippocampal volume in the association between emotional abuse and peer victimization in adolescents with major depressive disorder', *European Child & Adolescent Psychiatry*, 34, pp. 3175–3183. doi:10.1007/s00787-025-02737-2.

Lereya, S.T., Samara, M. and Wolke, D. (2013) 'Parenting behavior and the risk of becoming a victim and a bully/victim: A meta-analysis study', *Child Abuse & Neglect*, 37(12), pp. 1091–1108. doi:10.1016/j.chiabu.2013.03.001.

Morales-Hidalgo, P., Voltas, N. and Canals, J. (2024) 'Self-perceived bullying victimization in pre-adolescents on the autism spectrum: EPINED study', *Autism*, 28(11), pp. 2848–2857. doi:10.1177/13623613241244875.

National Institute for Health and Care Excellence (NICE) (2018) *Post-traumatic stress disorder (NG116)*. Available at: www.nice.org.uk/guidance/ng116 (Accessed: 1 March 2026).

National Institute for Health and Care Excellence (NICE) (2019) *Depression in children and young people: Identification and management (NG134)*. Available at: www.nice.org.uk/guidance/ng134 (Accessed: 1 March 2026).

National Institute for Health and Care Excellence (NICE) (2022) *Self-harm: Assessment, management and preventing recurrence (NG225)*. Available at: www.nice.org.uk/guidance/ng225 (Accessed: 1 March 2026).

Park, I., Kim, Y.S., Koh, Y.J., Leventhal, B.L. and Kim, Y.S. (2020) 'Prevalence of and factors associated with school bullying in students with autism spectrum disorder: A cross-cultural meta-analysis', *Yonsei Medical Journal*, 61(11), pp. 909–922. doi:10.3349/ymj.2020.61.11.909.

Shaheen, A.M., Hamdan, K.M., Albqoor, M., Othman, A.K., Amre, H.M. and Abu Hazeem, M.N. (2019) 'Perceived social support from family and friends and bullying victimization among adolescents', *Children and Youth Services Review*, 107, 104503. doi:10.1016/j.childyouth.2019.104503.

Stilwell, S.M., Scott, B.A., Murphy, H. and Lee, E. (2026) 'Affirm my identity, save my life: A scoping review of suicide prevention efforts for LGBTQ+ youth in K–12 schools', *School Mental Health*, 18(2), pp. 357–369. doi: 10.1007/s12310-025-09797-4.

Wallace, E.R., O'Neill, S. and Lagdon, S. (2024) 'Risk and protective factors for suicidality among lesbian, gay, bisexual, transgender, and queer (LGBTQ+) young people, from countries with a high global acceptance index (GAI), within the context of the socio-ecological model: A scoping review', *Journal of Adolescence*, 96, pp. 897–924. doi:10.1002/jad.12308.

Zhu, Y., Li, W., O'Brien, J.E. and Liu, T. (2021) 'Parent–child attachment moderates the associations between cyberbullying victimization and adolescents' health/mental health problems', *Journal of Interpersonal Violence*, 36(17–18), pp. NP9272–NP9298. doi:10.1177/0886260519854559.

Part III

Changing the System

Chapter 6

What Teachers Can Do to Prevent and Heal the Impact of Bullying

Abstract

Teachers occupy a pivotal position in both the prevention of bullying and the recovery of pupils affected by it. This chapter argues that effective school responses require more than identifying incidents and applying sanctions. Teachers need to understand how bullying can affect behaviour, learning, relationships and emotional regulation, and how these effects may present differently across pupils. Drawing on trauma-informed principles, the chapter explores how classroom routines, relational safety, emotional literacy and predictable boundaries can reduce harm and support recovery. It distinguishes between bullying prevention, which aims to shape school culture before harm occurs, and anti-bullying response, which addresses incidents once they arise. Particular attention is given to pupils with overlapping roles, including bully-victims, and to the specific vulnerabilities associated with prejudice-based bullying. The chapter also critically examines whole-school programmes such as KiVa and Olweus, arguing that structured interventions can be useful when implemented carefully, but should not be treated as universal solutions. Sustainable change depends on trained staff, consistent policy, pupil voice and a school culture in which safety and belonging are actively protected.

In This Chapter

- Why teachers play a crucial role in preventing bullying, responding to incidents and supporting recovery
- Why bullying should be understood as a group process that is shaped by power, status and peer dynamics, not simply as children falling out
- Which pupils may be more vulnerable to being targeted and how signs of vulnerability can be misunderstood
- How identity-based bullying, including racism, homophobia, ableism and other forms of prejudice, can deepen harm

DOI: 10.4324/9781003771777-10

- The difference between children who bully others, children who are bullied and children who are both
- What trauma-informed practice looks like in the classroom, and how it can support safety, regulation and trust
- How teachers can contribute to prevention, early intervention and whole-school change
- Why programmes such as KiVa and Olweus should be used cautiously and as part of a broader school strategy, rather than treated as universal solutions

Teachers are often the adults best placed to notice the early signs that a child is struggling. They see changes in attendance, confidence, behaviour, relationships and engagement with learning. For that reason, they are not simply witnesses to bullying. They are key actors in prevention, protection and recovery. This chapter examines what teachers can do at classroom and whole-school level to prevent bullying, respond effectively when it occurs, and support children whose sense of safety, identity and belonging has been damaged by peer harm.

The chapter also adopts a distinction that is often blurred in practice. Bullying prevention refers to the proactive work that reduces the likelihood of bullying taking root in school culture. The anti-bullying response refers to what adults do once bullying has occurred, including investigation, support, accountability, follow-up and repair. Both matter, but they require different forms of thinking, planning and professional judgement. The distinction is important because schools that focus only on incident response often miss the wider climate that allows harm to flourish, while schools that speak in general terms about kindness without robust response procedures may fail the pupils who most need protection.

Teachers as Agents of Prevention, Protection and Repair

Teachers influence bullying dynamics in at least three ways. First, they shape peer culture. Pupils learn quickly what is tolerated, what is ignored and what is taken seriously. If a teacher consistently challenges ridicule, exclusion and contempt, pupils receive a clear message that cruelty is not socially rewarded. Secondly, teachers act as protectors. Their willingness to notice, to ask and to follow up can interrupt a pattern of harm before it becomes entrenched. Thirdly, teachers support repair. When bullying has occurred, pupils often need more than reassurance that the incident has been logged. They need help to regain trust in adults, confidence in learning, and a sense that school can once again be a safe place.

This makes the classroom a significant site of intervention. While leadership, policy and safeguarding systems matter enormously, much of the daily reality of bullying is experienced within ordinary routines, lining up, group work, change rooms, corridor movement, online interactions that spill into lessons and subtle forms of status management between peers. Teachers therefore need a model of practice that joins pastoral awareness with evidence-informed action. This is not about asking teachers to become therapists. It is about recognising that emotionally attuned, structured and fair classroom practice can either buffer the effects of bullying or deepen them.

Current statutory guidance reinforces this responsibility. Department for Education guidance makes clear that schools should prevent and respond to bullying through their overall behaviour policy, while Keeping Children Safe in Education states that behaviour policy should include measures to prevent bullying, including cyberbullying, and prejudice-based and discriminatory bullying (Department for Education, 2021; Department for Education, 2025).

Recognising Bullying-related Distress in the Classroom

Not all pupils disclose bullying directly. Many communicate distress through behaviour, attendance, physical symptoms or social withdrawal. A child who once answered confidently may become quiet and avoid eye contact. Another may begin missing school with recurrent headaches or stomach aches. Some pupils become unusually vigilant, scanning the room for threat, avoiding certain classmates or asking repeatedly to leave the lesson. Others may present as irritable, defensive or aggressive in ways that are easily misread as simple defiance.

These responses are understandable when bullying is seen as a chronic threat to safety and belonging. A pupil who is repeatedly mocked, excluded, threatened or humiliated may start to anticipate danger even in relatively ordinary social situations. This can disrupt concentration, working memory, emotional regulation and trust. Teachers should therefore attend to patterns, not isolated behaviours. The question is rarely whether a child is perfectly calm and articulate enough to report bullying in a straightforward way. The more useful question is whether there has been a meaningful change in functioning that requires sensitive exploration.

Teachers can look for clusters of indicators, sudden friendship breakdown, reluctance to join group work, deterioration in school attendance, damaged belongings, repeated requests to sit near adults, visible fear around particular peers, tearfulness after transitions, and changes in academic confidence. None of these signs proves bullying on its own. However, when several occur together, especially alongside a shift in mood or participation, they warrant careful follow-up. Such follow-up should be private, calm and non-accusatory. Public questioning can increase shame and may reduce the likelihood of disclosure.

This is especially important because the mental health consequences of bullying are well documented. School bullying is associated with anxiety, depression, school disengagement and later psychological distress. In a longitudinal cohort study, bully-victims, children who are both targeted and aggressive towards others, showed particularly elevated mental health difficulties over time (Lereya et al., 2015). Teachers are therefore not merely identifying interpersonal conflict. In some cases, they are identifying one of the earliest visible markers of broader emotional harm.

Signs that Merit Follow-up

A sudden fall in participation, attendance or concentration.
Repeated physical complaints linked to school attendance, such as headaches or stomach aches.
Avoidance of specific peers, spaces or group activities.
Damaged belongings, visible anxiety or changes in mood after social transitions.
Increased reactivity, withdrawal or emotional shutdown without an obvious classroom explanation.

Why Pupils Do Not Always Disclose

Recognising distress is not the same as receiving a disclosure. One of the difficulties for teachers is that pupils who are being bullied do not always use the language adults expect. Some do not identify their experiences as bullying, especially when humiliation, exclusion, teasing, social manipulation or online harassment have gradually become normalised within the peer group. Others fear that reporting will make matters worse, either because retaliation is likely or because prior efforts to seek help have not led to meaningful protection. Shame also plays a powerful role. For some children, especially older pupils, acknowledging victimisation can feel socially dangerous because it appears to confirm the very loss of status that bullying has already created.

This helps explain why some of the most vulnerable pupils remain invisible for longer than teachers might expect. A child may present with recurrent physical complaints, emotional shutdown or irritability without ever making a direct allegation. Another may minimise what has happened with phrases such as 'it's nothing', 'we were just messing around', or 'they do it to everyone'. In these situations, the teacher's role is not to force disclosure, but to create the conditions in which disclosure becomes safer. That means a private conversation, careful listening and a willingness to return to the issue more than once. It also means noticing when a pupil appears relieved simply to have been seen. In practice, many children disclose indirectly before they disclose explicitly.

This challenge becomes even more significant when pupils occupy overlapping roles. Children who are both bullied and aggressive towards others often confuse adult interpretation because their distress is mixed with behaviours that attract sanction. A pupil who lashes out in class, argues with staff or behaves in controlling ways with peers may still be living with ongoing victimisation elsewhere in the school day. Haataja's implementation work is especially useful here because it showed that identifying long-term victimisation remained difficult even in schools using a structured anti-bullying programme. Teachers were more likely to miss chronically victimised pupils when those pupils did not disclose, when cases were socially complex, or when victimisation was entangled with other behavioural concerns (Haataja, 2016).

For teachers, the implication is important. Schools should not rely only on formal complaints if they want to identify bullying early. The sensitive monitoring of attendance, friendship changes, group work participation, break-time behaviour and repeated emotional disruption often provides the first indication that a child no longer feels safe. This is particularly true where pupils have communication differences, additional learning needs or limited confidence in adult response. In such cases, the question 'Has this child reported bullying?' may be less useful than 'What is this child's pattern of functioning telling us?'

A further reason pupils may not disclose is that they do not trust adult intervention. Children quickly form impressions about whether reporting is likely to lead to protection, minimisation or public exposure. If earlier incidents in the school have ended with vague reassurance, delayed action or pressure to 'be friends again', pupils may conclude that silence is the safer option. This is one reason why teacher consistency matters so much. Even children who are not directly involved in a case are watching how adults respond. They notice who is believed, who is dismissed, and whether cruelty carries social consequences.

Disclosure is therefore best understood as relational rather than purely procedural. Reporting systems matter, but they work best in schools where pupils already believe that adults will notice, listen and act proportionately. Teachers contribute to this belief in everyday ways. A child who has seen a teacher challenge mockery calmly, follow up concerns discreetly and protect dignity is more likely to speak when something is wrong. Conversely, a child who has seen adults laugh off humiliation or treat social harm as trivial may remain silent even when distress is severe.

Creating Trauma-informed Classrooms

Bullying does not only hurt feelings. It can activate the body's stress response and change the way pupils experience the school day. A trauma-informed approach is helpful here, not because every bullied child meets criteria for trauma-related disorder, but because trauma-informed practice offers a practical framework for responding to distress without increasing shame or threat. The Office for Health Improvement and Disparities defines trauma-informed practice as an approach grounded in the understanding that trauma can affect neurological, biological, psychological and social development, and identifies six key principles: safety, trust, choice, collaboration, empowerment and cultural consideration (Office for Health Improvement and Disparities, 2022).

In educational settings, trauma-informed practice means that teachers do not reduce distressed behaviour to character flaws. Instead, they ask what the behaviour might be communicating and what environmental support is needed. This does not mean removing boundaries. A trauma-informed classroom is not permissive. It is structured, predictable and relational. Pupils know what is expected of them, but they are also more likely to feel safe enough to meet those expectations because they are not being managed through fear, sarcasm or public humiliation.

Predictability matters. Visual routines, consistent transitions, clear instructions and calm adult responses reduce ambiguity, and ambiguity often fuels anxiety in children who already feel unsafe. Relational safety matters too. A pupil is more likely to disclose, repair and re-engage when they experience the teacher as fair, emotionally steady and non-judgemental. Emotional literacy also matters. When pupils are routinely given the language to recognise and name their feelings, they are better able to understand their own responses and seek help before distress escalates.

This has practical implications. Teachers can begin the day with a soft start, such as a calm entry task, quiet music, or a brief emotional check-in. They can provide access to regulation tools, such as fidget objects, breathing prompts and designated quiet spaces that do not carry punitive stigma. Corrections can be framed in language that protects dignity, for example, 'Let us reset that and try again respectfully', rather than 'You are being rude'. These are not cosmetic changes. They alter the emotional tone of the classroom and reduce the likelihood that ordinary moments of correction feel like further attack.

Practical Trauma-informed Classroom Moves

Use predictable routines and explicit transitions so that pupils know what is coming next.

Offer quiet regulation spaces or brief reset routines without labelling them as punishment.

Use private correction where possible, especially for pupils already carrying shame or social vulnerability.

Build in emotional literacy through check-ins, reflective prompts and respectful discussion.
Respond to escalation with calm containment first, then problem-solving once the pupil is regulated.

From Concern to Action: What Teachers Should Do Next

Trauma-informed practice is most useful when it informs action, not merely interpretation. Once a teacher becomes concerned that a pupil may be experiencing bullying, the next steps matter greatly. A calm, proportionate and well-documented response helps prevent two common errors: overreaction that exposes the pupil further, and underreaction that leaves the child feeling unprotected. Teachers are rarely the sole investigators of bullying, but they are often the first adults to begin the process that determines whether a concern is taken seriously.

The first task is to create a safe opening for communication. This should usually happen in private, away from peers, and at a time when the pupil is not already dysregulated. Questions need to be open enough to invite description without suggesting answers. A teacher might begin by naming the change they have noticed rather than assuming the cause. For example, 'I've noticed you seem less settled at lunch and quieter in group work. I wanted to check how things have been for you'. This kind of opening reduces pressure and avoids turning the conversation into an interrogation.

If the pupil does begin to talk, the teacher should focus first on listening rather than immediately problem-solving. Children often need to know that they have been believed before they can think clearly about what should happen next. It is also important not to promise secrecy that cannot be kept. A more careful and honest response is to explain that the information will only be shared with the people who need it in order to help keep the pupil safe. This maintains trust, while preserving safeguarding responsibilities.

Documentation is the next essential step. A concern that is only remembered informally is easy to minimise later, especially if the behaviour seems intermittent or takes relational rather than physical forms. Teachers should therefore make a factual record as soon as possible, noting what was observed, what the pupil said in their own words where relevant, when and where incidents appear to occur, who may be involved, and what immediate actions were taken. This is not bureaucratic overkill. Patterns of bullying often become visible only when separate small events are recorded and reviewed together.

The immediate response should then focus on safety. That may involve alerting pastoral staff, adjusting seating, changing group arrangements, increasing adult visibility at key transition points or quietly checking what happens at lunch or break, or in corridors, change rooms, transport or online spillover into the school day. Safety planning should be proportionate and discreet. Children are often sensitive to being singled out in ways that further damage status. Teachers therefore need to protect without pathologising. Small practical changes are often more effective than highly visible displays of concern.

At this stage, it is also worth distinguishing between support, accountability and resolution. Support means ensuring that the harmed pupil feels protected and emotionally held. Accountability means addressing the behaviour of the pupil or pupils who caused the harm. Resolution means a longer-term improvement in the child's sense of safety, belonging and functioning. These are related, but not identical. Schools sometimes move too quickly from incident recognition to a symbolic act of resolution, for example, an apology or brief meeting, without first ensuring that support and accountability have been handled well. Teachers can help prevent this by keeping the focus on what actually changes after the initial report.

Follow-up is critical. A pupil may disclose once and then retreat if nothing visible improves. Conversely, a pupil may say 'it's better now' simply because they are exhausted by adult attention or fear being seen as difficult. Teachers should therefore revisit the issue over time. The most useful follow-up questions are not only 'Has it stopped?', but also 'How are lessons feeling now?', 'Are break times any easier?', 'Do you know who to go to if it starts again?', and 'Is there anywhere in school that still feels difficult?' These questions recognise that recovery involves more than the absence of a new incident.

Teachers also need to communicate with colleagues in a way that supports coherence. If one member of staff responds with care and urgency, while another dismisses the behaviour as routine conflict, the pupil receives a confused and unsafe message. Strong schools reduce this risk by ensuring that concerns are passed on clearly, that reporting routes are understood, and that there is agreement about the language being used. Bullying, conflict, relational aggression, identity-based harassment and peer fall-out are not interchangeable terms. The more precise the professional language, the more coherent the response is likely to be.

Seen in this way, trauma-informed practice is not only about kindness. It is about disciplined, emotionally intelligent action. It requires teachers to notice, listen, record, protect, communicate and review. That is what turns pastoral concern into meaningful intervention.

What Teachers Must Avoid

If teachers are to prevent secondary harm, they need to know not only what to do, but what to avoid. Public shaming is one of the clearest risks. Calling out a distressed child in front of peers, using sarcasm, forcing a public apology or making examples of pupils may reproduce the powerlessness at the core of bullying. Trauma-informed guidance specifically warns against re-traumatisation, which can occur when an interaction echoes previous experiences of threat, humiliation or loss of control (Office for Health Improvement and Disparities, 2022).

Teachers should also avoid minimisation. Telling a child to ignore it, toughen up or stop being sensitive communicates that their experience is not credible. Equally problematic is over-simplifying harmful peer dynamics as 'falling out' when one pupil is being repeatedly targeted within a clear power imbalance. Such framing can shift the burden onto the harmed child to reconcile, compromise or display resilience without first ensuring safety. Another risk is assuming that every child who bullies is simply malicious. Some are, in fact, distressed pupils acting through status seeking, impulsivity, fear or learned aggression. That does not remove accountability, but it does mean that punitive reaction alone may be insufficient.

Supporting Recovery After Bullying

Stopping an incident is only the beginning. Many pupils continue to carry the after-effects of bullying long after the visible behaviour has ceased. They may fear that adults will not protect them, expect peers to reject them, or interpret neutral situations as signs of renewed threat. Some become academically cautious, avoiding speaking, taking risks or participating in public tasks for fear of drawing attention. Others remain socially isolated even after the original perpetrators have moved on.

Teachers can support recovery by rebuilding predictability, competence and belonging. This may include flexible deadlines for pupils whose concentration has been impaired, alternative ways of demonstrating learning, carefully planned seating arrangements, and regular check-ins that ask not only about work completion, but about how safe and included the pupil feels. Simple acts of attunement matter. Greeting a child by name, noticing effort, pairing them with emotionally safe peers, and ensuring they are not repeatedly left on the margins of classroom collaboration can all contribute to repair.

Recovery also depends on coordination. A child who has experienced sustained bullying may need support that extends beyond one classroom. Teachers should therefore work with pastoral staff, special educational needs coordinators, safeguarding leads, school counsellors and families where appropriate. A strong response includes monitoring over time. It is not enough to ask whether the original incident has stopped. Staff should ask whether attendance, learning confidence, peer relationships and emotional presentation are improving. Without this follow-up, schools may overestimate resolution and underestimate the lingering effects of peer harm.

Case Example 1: The Withdrawn Pupil

A Year 6 pupil who was previously lively and engaged begins to arrive late, avoids reading aloud and asks to stay in at break. No direct disclosure is made. A trauma-informed teacher notices the change, checks in privately, and learns that the pupil has been excluded from a friendship group and mocked online after school. Rather than treating the behaviour as lack of effort, the teacher adjusts classroom participation expectations temporarily, liaises with pastoral staff, ensures supervised safety at unstructured times, and builds the pupil back into learning through supported small-group work. The response is protective because it joins investigation with recovery support rather than treating disclosure as the end point.

Understanding Bully-victims and Complex Peer Roles

One of the most important corrections to simplistic anti-bullying discourse is the recognition that some pupils are both targeted and aggressive. These bully-victims do not fit neatly into a binary of victim and perpetrator. They may be victimised by some peers, while intimidating others, or they may oscillate between vulnerability and aggression, depending on the context. This group is especially important because it is often associated with more severe social and emotional difficulties than either victims or perpetrators alone (Lereya et al., 2015).

For teachers, this complexity matters. If a child who has disclosed bullying later lashes out at others, staff may be tempted to see the original disclosure as exaggerated or manipulative. Equally, when a pupil is known to act aggressively, adults may miss the fact that the same pupil is being humiliated or excluded elsewhere. Both errors can deepen harm. Children in overlapping roles often need support that combines accountability, emotional regulation, close supervision and skilled relationship work. They may require help

Box 6.1 What Teachers Must Avoid

Public shaming, sarcasm or calling pupils out in front of their peers.
Treating repeated bullying as ordinary conflict or a simple disagreement.
Insisting on immediate reconciliation before safety has been restored.
Telling pupils to ignore it, grow a thicker skin, or solve it themselves.
Focusing only on sanctions without understanding the wider peer dynamics and the needs of both harmed and harming pupils.

understanding their own responses to threat, learning alternative ways of gaining status or protection, and repairing the damage they have caused without losing access to support themselves.

Recent classroom-level evidence shows that teacher interventions have distinct effects on bullying-related roles. Burger et al. (2022) found that disciplinary sanctions were associated with the reduced likelihood of being a bully or victim, group discussion increased the likelihood of pupils becoming defenders, and increased teacher non-intervention was associated with a greater likelihood of victimisation and a lower likelihood of defender behaviour over time. These findings are useful because they challenge the idea that any teacher response will do. Different responses shape different peer roles, and non-intervention is not neutral. It communicates permission to the peer group.

Case Example 2: The Bully-victim in a High-conflict Classroom

A Year 8 pupil is repeatedly sanctioned for making hostile comments and pushing in corridors. Staff initially describe him as the problem. However, closer examination reveals that he is also being goaded, filmed and excluded by older boys during lunch and online. A narrow disciplinary response would address only visible aggression. A better response holds him accountable for the harm he has caused, while also addressing his own victimisation, regulating his timetable during high-risk periods, and involving pastoral staff in a coordinated plan. This approach neither excuses harm nor abandons the child to it. It recognises that some pupils need protection and accountability at the same time.

Addressing the Pupil Who has Caused Harm Without Reinforcing Shame

Where a pupil has engaged in bullying behaviour, teachers face a difficult balance. They must be clear that the behaviour is unacceptable, but they also need to avoid responses that escalate defensiveness, humiliation or retaliation. This is especially important in cases involving repeated aggression, status seeking or complex bully-victim roles. A weak response risks communicating tolerance, while a shaming response may harden the child's self-protective stance without producing genuine change.

Recent evidence helps sharpen this point. Garandeau et al. (2016) examined how pupils who had bullied others perceived staff intervention discussions. Their findings are particularly useful for teachers because they distinguish between condemning the behaviour and blaming the child. Attempts to arouse empathy for the victim and clear condemnation of the bullying behaviour were both associated with greater intention to stop. By contrast, blaming the child had no significant effect. Intention to change was highest when empathy arousal and condemnation of the behaviour were both strong. This does not mean that teachers should avoid firmness. It means that firmness is more effective when directed at the behaviour, and paired with a clear moral and relational message about its impact.

This distinction is practical, not merely theoretical. Saying 'What you did was cruel, it caused harm, and it must stop', is very different from saying 'You are a bully, this is just who you are'. The first communicates accountability and possibility. The second risks fixing the child inside a morally contaminated identity that may invite either collapse or further oppositional behaviour. In school contexts, where reputation and status already matter intensely, adult language can either interrupt or intensify those dynamics.

This is also where the findings from Burger et al. (2022) are helpful. Their classroom-level work suggests that teacher responses shape peer roles over time. Disciplinary sanctions were associated with the reduced likelihood of being a bully or victim, group discussion increased the likelihood of pupils adopting defender roles, and teacher non-intervention was associated with greater victimisation and lower defender behaviour. Taken together, these studies suggest that adult action matters, but the form of that action matters as well. Neither passive observation nor indiscriminate punishment is enough on its own.

For classroom teachers, several implications follow. First, harmful behaviour should be named clearly and early. Ambiguous language is rarely effective in cases of repeated aggression or humiliation because it leaves too much room for social reinterpretation within the peer group. Secondly, the child who has caused harm should be helped to understand the impact of what they have done, not simply the fact that they have broken a rule. This is where perspective-taking and empathy work matter. Thirdly, accountability should include restoration where appropriate, but not in ways that rush the harmed pupil into contact or reconciliation before safety has been established.

It is also worth recognising that the pupil who has caused harm may be using aggression instrumentally. For some children, bullying functions as a route to status, group belonging, protection from their own victimisation or discharge of dysregulated emotion. A teacher response that focuses only on punishment may suppress behaviour temporarily without changing the conditions that made it useful to the child in the first place. Effective intervention therefore requires a dual lens. The school must protect others from harm, but it must also ask what needs to change if the pupil is to behave differently over time.

In practice, this may involve structured follow-up conversations, social and emotional coaching, increased adult monitoring, work on perspective-taking, careful scrutiny of peer group reinforcements and, where relevant, wider pastoral or family involvement. For some pupils, particularly those who are also being targeted elsewhere, the task is not merely to 'stop bullying', but to find alternative ways of gaining recognition, managing threat and participating in peer life without using domination as a defence.

A sophisticated school response therefore rejects two simplifications at once. It rejects the idea that kindness alone will stop harmful behaviour, and rejects the idea that blame alone creates change. Teachers need a more precise formulation: condemn the behaviour, protect the harmed pupil, build empathy where possible, and avoid shaming the child into a fixed identity. That is not softness. It is disciplined, evidence-informed practice.

Responding to Identity-based and Prejudice-based Bullying

Bullying is not experienced uniformly. Some pupils are targeted because of disability, race, religion, class, body size, appearance, care experience, sexuality, gender expression or other stigmatised aspects of identity. This matters because identity-based bullying often draws power from wider social inequalities rather than from a single interpersonal conflict. It is therefore both a peer issue and a cultural issue. Teachers need to understand that harm can be intensified when bullying targets who a child is, or is perceived to be, rather than simply what they do.

Keeping Children Safe in Education explicitly identifies prejudice-based and discriminatory bullying as requiring preventive measures within behaviour policy (Department for Education, 2025). Recent research also shows that teachers' responses to identity-based bullying are shaped by teacher and school characteristics, including training, school support and wider diversity conditions. In a UK study of 422 educators, Görzig et al. (2026) found that teacher-level and school-level factors influenced responses such as perceived seriousness, empathy, responsibility and the likelihood of intervention. This is important because it suggests that good intentions are not enough. Schools need specific training and supportive conditions if staff are to respond consistently and equitably.

Teachers therefore need guidance that goes beyond generic advice to be kind or inclusive. They need to recognise racist bullying, disablist bullying, sexist bullying, and homophobic, biphobic or transphobic bullying when they occur. They need the confidence to name such behaviour accurately, record it consistently and challenge it without defensiveness or minimisation. Identity-specific prevention also involves curriculum representation, explicit anti-prejudice teaching, consultation with pupils about where they feel unsafe, and the use of data to detect patterns across year groups, spaces and pupil groups. This is where anti-bullying work intersects with safeguarding, equality duties and school ethos.

Identity-specific Strategies for Schools

Train staff to recognise prejudice-based forms of bullying, not only overt physical or verbal incidents.
Record identity-based incidents accurately and review patterns termly.
Ensure curriculum materials represent diverse pupils with dignity rather than tokenism.
Consult pupils and families about where exclusion and humiliation are most likely to occur.
Link anti-bullying work to safeguarding, equality, attendance and pastoral systems rather than treating it as an isolated theme week.

Identity, Belonging, Attendance and the Online Spillover

Identity-based bullying is particularly damaging because it attacks not only a child's social position in school, but also their sense of legitimacy and belonging. A pupil who is repeatedly targeted because of race, disability, religion, sexuality, gender expression, body size, poverty or perceived difference is receiving a message about who is allowed to belong safely and who is not. For that reason, teachers need to understand identity-based bullying not only as misconduct between pupils, but as a threat to equal participation in school life.

One consequence is that attendance can become a disguised indicator of harm. Children do not always say, 'I am being bullied because of who I am.' Instead, they may start arriving late, requesting to go home, avoiding particular subjects or spaces, or developing patterns of absence that appear inconsistent until viewed through the lens of social safety. For some pupils, especially those from groups already used to misunderstanding or stigma, school refusal is not simply anxiety in the abstract. It may be a rational response to repeated exposure to humiliation. Teachers therefore need to ask what attendance is communicating, particularly when emotional distress, isolation or visible discomfort around specific peer groups accompanies it.

Belonging is equally important. Anti-bullying practice often focuses heavily on stopping overt incidents, but pupils recover more fully when schools also rebuild inclusion. A child who is no longer openly mocked may still feel peripheral, watched or symbolically marked as different. Teachers can address this by thinking carefully about participation structures. Who is repeatedly chosen last in group activities? Who is always positioned as the object of curiosity, pity or token celebration? Who has to endure jokes that others are permitted to frame as harmless? These are not separate from bullying. They are often the culture in which bullying thrives.

This is one reason curriculum and representation matter. Pupils are safer where the wider environment communicates that human difference is ordinary, respected and not a licence for degradation. However, representation on its own is not enough. Children notice very quickly whether adults can actually name prejudice when it occurs. A school may celebrate diversity symbolically, yet still fail pupils if staff are hesitant, defensive or inconsistent when confronted with racist, disablist, sexist or homophobic conduct. Teachers therefore need language, confidence and institutional backing, not only good intentions.

Identity-based bullying also frequently has an online dimension. Even when incidents begin in school, they may continue through messaging, group chats, image sharing, social exclusion on platforms, or after-school commentary that returns to the classroom the next morning. Teachers cannot control all digital life, but they can recognise that children's online and offline worlds are rarely separate. A pupil who has been humiliated online overnight may arrive at school already dysregulated, ashamed or expecting further exposure. This means that staff should not assume that bullying has 'left school' simply because the latest incident occurred on a device at home. Where online behaviour materially affects a child's safety, participation or treatment in school, it becomes part of the educational and safeguarding picture.

Family partnership is particularly important here. Parents and carers may notice avoidance, distress, sleep disruption, device anxiety or reluctance to attend school before teachers have seen a full pattern. At the same time, some families, especially those who have themselves experienced discrimination, may be understandably sceptical about whether the school will respond fairly. Initial communication therefore matters a great deal. Families need to hear that the concern has been understood, that identity-based harm will be named accurately rather than diluted into generic 'unkindness', and that the school has a plan for both immediate protection and follow-up.

Teachers can support this process by being precise and evidence-led. It is better to say 'Your child has described repeated comments about disability and exclusion from group work; we are treating this as a bullying concern with a prejudice-based element and are putting support in place', than to rely on vague reassurance. Precision communicates seriousness. It also reduces the risk that the family experiences the school as evasive or minimising.

Ultimately, responding well to identity-based bullying requires more than sensitivity. It requires institutional clarity about safety, equality, attendance and participation. The question is not only whether overt incidents are reduced. It is whether the child can move through school without being repeatedly reminded that difference makes them fair game for humiliation. Teachers play an important role in that everyday reality because they are the adults most likely to see how belonging is either protected or eroded in real time.

Whole-school Prevention, Anti-Bullying Response and School Culture

Although this chapter centres teachers, classroom action is only part of the picture. Lasting change requires a whole-school approach. Government guidance states that schools should take action to prevent and respond to bullying as part of their overall behaviour policy (Department for Education, 2021). More recent statutory safeguarding guidance repeats that behaviour policy should include measures to prevent bullying, including cyberbullying, and prejudice-based and discriminatory bullying (Department for Education, 2025). This makes anti-bullying work a matter of institutional responsibility rather than optional pastoral preference.

A whole-school approach includes clear definitions of bullying, staff confidence in recognising different forms of harm, multiple reporting routes, reliable recording, a regular review of hotspots and trends, and visible adult presence in higher-risk contexts such as corridors, playgrounds, lunch spaces and changing areas. It also includes pupil voice. Children often know long before adults which spaces are unsafe, which jokes are functioning as harassment, and which social hierarchies are driving exclusion. Schools that do not ask pupils what school feels like from their perspective may miss precisely the information they most need.

Whole-school climate matters because bullying does not arise in a vacuum. Research on authoritative school climate suggests that students fare better in schools characterised by both supportive adult relationships and fair, consistent discipline. Cornell and Huang (2016) found that schools with a more authoritative climate had lower levels of bullying, fighting, weapon carrying, substance use, and suicidal thoughts and behaviour. This does not mean that climate solves everything. It means that pupils are more likely to thrive where warmth and structure coexist, and where adult authority is experienced as fair rather than arbitrary.

The wider literature on whole-school approaches also points to potential value, while remaining clear about limitations. A 2025 Oxford literature review on whole-school approaches to wellbeing concluded that such models can support mental health, social and emotional learning, and school climate, but also noted that effects are often small to moderate and highly dependent on implementation, participation and school context (Zhou et al., 2025). For bullying, this is a crucial point. A whole-school approach is not a slogan. It is sustained organisational work.

Evidence-informed Programmes, with Caution

Schools often look to named programmes for structure and reassurance. This is understandable. A well-designed programme can provide shared language, staff training, lesson materials and clearer pathways for responding to incidents. However, the strongest conclusion from the recent literature is not that any one programme will work equally well in all schools, for all pupils, or across all outcomes. Rather, structured programmes can support prevention and response when they fit the school context, are implemented consistently, and are sustained over time. Recent review work suggests that anti-bullying interventions can reduce bullying in schools, but it also emphasises that fit, feasibility and successful implementation remain under-studied, especially over the longer term and across different school contexts. The same review also notes a significant limitation in the evidence base, namely that few studies have examined whether programme effectiveness varies across racial, ethnic, sexual orientation, gender or socioeconomic groups (George et al., 2024).

KiVa, developed in Finland, remains one of the best-known anti-bullying programmes and is grounded in the idea that bullying is sustained by peer group processes and the social rewards gained from bystanders. The recent UK multicentre cluster randomised controlled trial offers the strongest current evidence for KiVa in this context. Across 118 primary schools and 11 111 pupils, Bowes et al. (2024) found that KiVa reduced student-reported bullying victimisation, with odds of victimisation 13 percent lower than in schools continuing with usual practice. Pupils in KiVa schools also showed higher empathy and fewer peer problems. However, the same trial found no differences in bullying perpetration, school-related happiness or broader emotional and behavioural problems, and no differences by gender or socioeconomic gradient. KiVa should therefore be presented as a promising and evidence-informed whole-school model, not as a universal remedy (Bowes et al., 2024).

It is also important to recognise that evidence from mainstream schools does not automatically transfer to all settings. This is particularly relevant for pupils with special educational needs and disabilities, who are often at increased risk of victimisation and may require adapted teaching, communication and reporting approaches. Badger et al. (2023) note that there is currently a lack of evidence-based anti-bullying programmes designed for special schools. In their pilot of KiVa SEND, two adapted KiVa lessons were co-developed and trialled in two English special schools, one supporting pupils with autism and one supporting pupils with severe and complex learning disabilities. Engagement from pupils and staff was high, the materials were considered acceptable, and the authors concluded that further development and formal testing were warranted. This is an important reminder that evidence-based programmes may need thoughtful adaptation, rather than simple transfer, when used with more diverse learning needs and communication profiles (Badger et al., 2023).

Olweus remains historically important as one of the earliest and most influential whole-school bullying prevention models. Its emphasis on school-wide rules, adult visibility, classroom meetings and parent engagement has shaped the field significantly. Yet evidence on its effectiveness has been mixed. In a controlled trial in public middle schools, Bauer et al. (2007) found some mixed positive effects that varied by subgroup, but no overall effect. More recent work suggests that implementation fidelity and teacher engagement matter greatly for outcomes. This is not an argument for abandoning structured programmes, but for resisting simplistic claims that named programmes guarantee success regardless of context.

The wider evidence base supports guarded optimism. The 2021 Campbell systematic review and meta-analysis concluded that school-based anti-bullying programmes reduce both perpetration and victimisation overall, but effect sizes are modest, and heterogeneity between studies is substantial (Gaffney et al., 2021). This is precisely the nuance schools need. Programmes can help, and some are worthwhile, but improvement depends on fit, fidelity, leadership, staff buy-in and sustained implementation. A weak school culture will not be repaired by a branded package alone.

Additional implementation research helps explain why caution is necessary when discussing named programmes. Haataja's work on KiVa implementation found that larger reductions in victimisation were achieved in classrooms where teachers showed higher adherence to the curriculum and spent more time preparing lessons, whereas bullying perpetration was not equally affected by implementation level. The same body of work also showed that sustained implementation was supported by principal backing and teacher belief in the programme, while the recognition of chronically victimised pupils remained a serious challenge. In schools beginning implementation, only around a quarter of long-term victims were recognised by staff, especially when pupils did not disclose their experiences or were also bullying others. More recent work on shared anti-bullying practices similarly found variation both within and between schools, and linked stronger perceptions of shared practice to professional role, school size, school wellbeing values, leadership promoting wellbeing and the use of a manualised programme. Together, these findings suggest that programme effectiveness depends not only on programme design, but also on leadership, preparation, staff buy-in and collective consistency across the school (Haataja, 2016; Sainio et al., 2026).

Named programmes can provide a valuable framework, but they are not substitutes for a healthy school culture. The wider evidence supports guarded optimism, not overstatement. Whole-school approaches appear more promising than fragmented or purely classroom-based efforts, but improvement depends on fit, fidelity, leadership, staff commitment and sustained implementation. Programmes can help, but they work best when embedded within a broader school commitment to safety, belonging and a consistent adult response.

Relational and Restorative Work in School Response

Alongside whole-school programmes, some schools use restorative approaches to reduce reliance on exclusionary discipline and improve relationships. Restorative practice is not a synonym for making pupils apologise or forcing mediated conversations immediately after harm. At its best, it is a relational framework that seeks accountability, understanding and repair, while preserving dignity. Gregory et al. (2015) found that teachers implementing restorative practices more strongly were viewed more positively by students and issued fewer exclusionary discipline referrals. The significance for bullying work is that relational repair and fair accountability are not opposites. They can be complementary when used carefully.

However, restorative approaches need boundaries. They should not be used in ways that pressure harmed pupils into confronting those who bullied them before they feel safe, nor should they replace protective action where there is ongoing intimidation or a serious power imbalance. Teachers need judgement here. Some situations require immediate separation, formal investigation and safeguarding escalation. Others may later benefit from a restorative process once safety has been secured. Restorative work should therefore be understood as one possible component of an anti-bullying response, not a blanket solution.

What Implementation Actually Requires From Schools

One of the clearest messages from the programme literature is that implementation is not a technical afterthought. It is often the difference between a school having a programme on paper and a school changing pupil experience in practice. This point matters because schools are often attracted to named interventions precisely because they appear to simplify anti-bullying work. In reality, the evidence suggests the opposite. Structured programmes may provide a framework, but they still demand leadership, staff coherence, preparation time, follow-through and adaptation to local conditions.

The recent UK KiVa trial is instructive here. Its results were promising, but measured. KiVa reduced student-reported victimisation and improved some peer-related outcomes, but effects were not universal across all outcomes, and the authors themselves emphasised caution and replication. That is not a weakness of the trial. It is exactly the kind of realistic evidence schools need. It tells us that programmes can help, but not that they eliminate the need for professional judgement, contextual fit or sustained organisational effort (Bowes et al., 2024).

Haataja's work on KiVa implementation deepens this further. It suggests that stronger reductions in victimisation were seen where teachers adhered more closely to the curriculum, prepared lessons more carefully and maintained implementation quality over time. The same work also showed how difficult it can be for staff to identify long-term victims, especially when pupils do not disclose or where victimisation is socially complex. In other words, even with a structured programme in place, schools still depend on adult attentiveness, consistency and willingness to engage seriously with what is actually happening in peer groups (Haataja, 2016).

This has major implications for teacher training and leadership. A school cannot reasonably expect anti-bullying work to be effective if staff have not been given time to understand the model, discuss likely barriers, practise difficult conversations, and agree how incidents will be recorded and followed up. Implementation is relational as well as procedural. Teachers need to know not only what the programme materials say, but how those materials connect to ordinary classroom life, transition points, safeguarding responsibilities and the realities of children whose distress does not arrive in neat categories.

The SEND adaptation literature reinforces this point. Badger et al. (2023) show that even a strong evidence-based programme may require careful co-development before it becomes suitable for special school settings. Their KiVa-SEND pilot found high engagement and perceived acceptability, but it also emphasised the need for further development and formal testing. This is a valuable corrective to the assumption that evidence transfers unchanged across contexts. Pupils with different communication needs, cognitive profiles and patterns of social vulnerability may require materials, examples, pacing and reporting processes that look quite different from those used in mainstream settings.

It follows that schools should think of implementation as a cycle rather than a launch event. A programme begins with an introduction, but it becomes meaningful only through repeated review. Staff need to know whether lessons are actually being delivered, whether pupils understand the content, whether reporting routes are being used, whether acute cases are being handled according to guidance, and whether the pupils most at risk are experiencing greater safety. This kind of implementation thinking is reflected in newer programme development work, which has moved increasingly toward assessing fidelity, staff attitudes, lesson quality and the handling of acute cases rather than assuming that delivery alone is enough.

The key analytical point is this: programme adoption is not the same as programme enactment. A school may purchase materials, schedule lessons, and still fall short if staff are unconvinced, stretched or inconsistent. Conversely, a school with a modest resource base may achieve more if leadership is strong, expectations are shared, and anti-bullying work is treated as part of the school's core moral and pastoral function rather than as an add-on. That is why a weak school culture cannot be repaired by branding alone. Programmes work best where adults act as a coherent community.

Teachers are central to this coherence. They are the people who translate institutional intention into lived pupil experience. They decide whether language in a lesson is connected to what happens in corridors and group work. They decide whether a disclosure is handled with seriousness or minimised. They decide whether dignity is protected during correction and whether follow-up actually happens. For that reason, implementation should not be discussed as something external to teaching. It is part of teaching. A whole-school anti-bullying strategy lives or fails in the accumulated quality of adult responses.

This is also why programme evaluation should include more than incident counts. Schools need to ask whether pupils feel safer reporting, whether staff are using common language, whether higher-risk groups are being protected effectively, and whether harmed pupils are genuinely recovering rather than simply becoming quieter. When implementation is understood in this richer way, evidence-informed practice becomes less about selecting the right package and more about building the conditions under which any good package can actually work.

From Classroom Action to Policy and Practice

For teachers to succeed, they need more than personal goodwill. They need training, time, reporting systems and leadership support. Schools should be able to answer several practical questions with clarity. What definition of bullying is used in the setting, and is it understood consistently by pupils and staff? How can pupils report concerns confidentially? Who follows up, within what timescale, and how is communication with families handled? How are repeat incidents tracked? Where are the school's hotspots, and which groups are most at risk? Which staff have received training in trauma-informed practice, identity-based bullying and effective intervention strategies?

These questions move anti-bullying work from aspiration to implementation. They also help bridge the gap between individual teacher effort and whole-school responsibility. A school can have caring teachers and still fail pupils if procedures are inconsistent or if repeated concerns disappear into weak recording systems. Equally, a school can have a strong policy on paper, and still fail if daily adult responses are dismissive or uneven. Meaningful change requires this dual emphasis. Systems matter, and so do relationships.

Questions Schools should be Able to Answer Clearly

How do pupils report bullying, and do they trust the process?
How are incidents recorded, reviewed and followed up over time?
What training do staff receive on trauma-informed practice and identity-based bullying?
How are families involved in prevention and response?
How does the school know whether harmed pupils are actually recovering, rather than simply becoming quieter?

Conclusion

Teachers cannot eliminate bullying on their own, but they can profoundly influence whether it is ignored, interrupted or healed. Their words, routines, relationships and judgements shape what pupils learn about power, safety and belonging every day. A child who is bullied may never remember the exact wording of a behaviour policy, but they are likely to remember whether a teacher noticed, believed them, protected them, and helped them recover.

The most effective teacher response is therefore neither purely punitive nor naively permissive. It is relational, structured and evidence-informed. It combines high expectations with safety, clear boundaries with dignity, and whole-school systems with human attunement. When teachers are supported to work in this way, classrooms become more than places where bullying is managed after the fact. They become places where children learn that cruelty is not normal, silence is not required, and recovery is possible.

Key Takeaways

- Bullying prevention is proactive work that shapes culture before harm occurs; anti-bullying response is what schools do once bullying has been identified
- Teachers are often the first adults to notice bullying-related distress through changes in behaviour, attendance, confidence and peer relationships
- Trauma-informed classrooms combine structure with emotional safety; they do not remove boundaries, but avoid shame and re-traumatisation
- Bully-victims require especially careful support because they may need protection and accountability at the same time
- Identity-based bullying demands explicit recognition, accurate recording and staff training; generic messages about kindness are not enough
- Whole-school approaches and named programmes can help, but outcomes depend on implementation quality, context and staff commitment rather than programme labels alone

References

Badger, J.R., Bowes, L., Salmivalli, C. and Hastings, R.P. (2023) 'Adapting an anti-bullying programme for UK special schools', *Support for Learning*, 38, pp. 178–182. Available at: https://doi.org/10.1111/1467-9604.12457.

Bauer, N.S., Lozano, P. and Rivara, F.P. (2007) 'The effectiveness of the Olweus Bullying Prevention Program in public middle schools: A controlled trial', *Journal of Adolescent Health*, 40(3), pp. 266–274.

Bowes, L., Babu, M., Badger, J.R., Broome, M.R., Cannings-John, R., Clarkson, S., Coulman, E., Edwards, R.T., Ford, T., Hastings, R.P., Hayes, R., Lugg-Widger, F., Owen-Jones, E., Patterson, P., Segrott, J., Sydenham, M., Townson, J., Watkins, R.C., Whiteley, H., Williams, M.E., Hutchings, J. and the Stand Together Team (2024) 'The effects and costs of an anti-bullying programme (KiVa) in UK primary schools: A multicentre cluster randomised controlled trial', *Psychological Medicine*, 54, pp. 4362–4373. doi: 10.1017/S0033291724002666.

Burger, C., Strohmeier, D. and Kollerová, L. (2022) 'Teachers can make a difference in bullying: Effects of teacher interventions on students' adoption of bully, victim, bully-victim or defender roles across time', *Journal of Youth and Adolescence*, 51, pp. 2312–2327. doi: 10.1007/s10964-022-01674-6.

Cornell, D. and Huang, F. (2016) 'Authoritative school climate and high school student risk behavior: A cross-sectional multi-level analysis of student self-reports', *Journal of Youth and Adolescence*, 45(11), pp. 2246–2259. doi: 10.1007/s10964-016-0424-3.

Department for Education (2021) *Preventing and tackling bullying: Advice for headteachers, staff and governing bodies*. London: Department for Education.

Department for Education (2025) *Keeping children safe in education 2025*. London: Department for Education.

Gaffney, H., Farrington, D.P. and Ttofi, M.M. (2021) 'Effectiveness of school-based programs to reduce bullying perpetration and victimization: An updated systematic review and meta-analysis', *Campbell Systematic Reviews*, 17(2), e1143. doi: 10.1002/cl2.1143.

Garandeau, C.F., Vartio, A., Poskiparta, E. and Salmivalli, C. (2016) 'School bullies' intention to change behavior following teacher interventions: Effects of empathy arousal, condemning of bullying, and blaming of the perpetrator', *Prevention Science*, 17, pp. 1034–1043. doi: 10.1007/s11121-016-0712-x.

George, P., Cosgrove, J., Taylor, J., Rao, N., Marshall, T., Ghose, S.S. and Patel, N.A. (2024) 'Antibullying interventions in schools: Assessing the evidence base', *Psychiatric Services*, 75(9), pp. 908–920. Available at: https://doi.org/10.1176/appi.ps.20230541.

Görzig, A., Betts, L.R., Maunder, R., Monks, C.P., De Amicis, L. and Bennett, S. (2026) 'Teachers' responses to identity-based bullying: Social inequality, identity, and diversity at teacher and school level', *International Journal of Bullying Prevention*, 8, pp. 83–102. doi: 10.1007/s42380-024-00281-2.

Gregory, A., Clawson, K., Davis, A. and Gerewitz, J. (2015) 'The promise of restorative practices to transform teacher-student relationships and achieve equity in school discipline', *Journal of Educational and Psychological Consultation*, 25(4), pp. 325–353. doi: 10.1080/10474412.2014.929950.

Haataja, A. (2016) *Implementing the KiVa antibullying program: What does it take?* Doctoral thesis. University of Turku. Turun Yliopiston Julkaisuja, Annales Universitatis Turkuensis, Ser. B, Tom. 420.

Lereya, S.T., Copeland, W.E., Zammit, S. and Wolke, D. (2015) 'Bully/victims: A longitudinal, population-based cohort study of their mental health', *European Child and Adolescent Psychiatry*, 24, pp. 1461–1471. doi: 10.1007/s00787-015-0705-5.

Office for Health Improvement and Disparities (2022) *Working definition of trauma-informed practice*. London: Department of Health and Social Care.

Sainio, M., Herkama, S., Torppa, M., Aro, T. and Hämeenaho, P. (2026) 'What explains the perception of having shared practices among school staff for anti-bullying work?', *International Journal of Bullying Prevention*, 8, pp. 7–19. doi: 10.1007/s42380-024-00271-4.

Zhou, W., Taylor, L., Boyle, L., Funk, S., DeBorst, L. and De Neve, J.-E. (2025) *Whole school approach to wellbeing in childhood and adolescence: Literature review*. Oxford: Wellbeing Research Centre, University of Oxford, in association with the International Baccalaureate Organization.

Chapter 7

Recovery, Clinical Formulation and Long-term Outcomes

Abstract

Recovery from bullying is not a simple return to baseline. For many children and adolescents, repeated peer victimisation disrupts emotional regulation, social expectations, behaviour and the sense of self, with effects that may persist well beyond the immediate bullying context. This chapter argues that recovery is best understood as a multi-level process involving neural, emotional, behavioural and social repair. Drawing on recent neurobiological, developmental and clinical literature, it examines how bullying-related stress may alter reward processing, social pain, threat sensitivity and cognitive control, while also shaping rumination, emotional reactivity and biased threat interpretation. Particular attention is given to bully-victims, whose presentations often combine trauma, aggression, anger dysregulation and poor social support. The chapter outlines how health and mental health professionals can assess bullying more effectively, use multi-informant and trauma-informed formulations, coordinate with schools and families, and select interventions that address both symptom reduction and long-term resilience. Recovery is presented not as symptom suppression alone, but as the rebuilding of safety, agency, connection and developmental possibility.

In This Chapter

- Why recovery from bullying involves neural, emotional, behavioural and social repair
- How bullying can act as a developmental stressor rather than a minor interpersonal difficulty
- How peer victimisation may shape threat sensitivity, rumination, emotional reactivity and later mental health
- Why bully-victims may present with complex patterns of trauma, anger, aggression and social rejection
- How health and mental health professionals can assess bullying using trauma-informed and multi-informant approaches

DOI: 10.4324/9781003771777-11

- How clinical formulation can move practice beyond simple victim labelling
- Why different presentations may require different recovery plans
- Why coordinated work between clinicians, families, schools and wider systems is essential
- How bullying can affect longer-term educational, psychosocial, economic and developmental outcomes
- What the evidence means for healthcare, mental health practice, family work and cross-sector collaboration

Recovery after bullying is often misunderstood as the disappearance of visible distress. In practice, recovery is more complex than that. A child may stop crying, return to school or appear outwardly calmer, while still expecting humiliation, anticipating rejection or remaining physiologically primed for threat. For health and mental health professionals, the task is therefore not only to identify distress, but to understand the mechanisms through which bullying becomes biologically and psychologically embedded, and the processes through which healing becomes possible.

Bullying should be conceptualised as a form of repeated interpersonal stress, which occurs during sensitive developmental periods. This matters because the developing brain is not simply reacting to isolated incidents. It is learning from patterns of danger, social exclusion, unpredictability and powerlessness. Recent neuroimaging evidence suggests that peer victimisation is associated with altered activation in systems involved in reward processing, social pain, affect regulation, social evaluation and cognitive control (Ke et al., 2022). Importantly, the evidence base remains methodologically mixed, with a strong reliance on cross-sectional designs and broad developmental age ranges. For that reason, claims about direct and uniform structural damage should be avoided. A more defensible interpretation is that repeated peer victimisation is associated with the altered neurodevelopmental processing of threat, reward, rejection and social belonging, which may help explain the persistence of anxiety, depression, withdrawal, irritability and risk-taking over time.

This more cautious framing is clinically useful. It allows practitioners to move beyond simplistic statements such as 'bullying changes the brain' and instead ask more precise questions. Has the young person become hypervigilant to social threat. Do they now misread ambiguity as danger. Are they repeatedly drawn back into distressing thoughts about humiliation, exclusion or retaliation. Are they over-controlled, emotionally flooded or oscillating between the two. These questions move assessment away from surface behaviour and towards mechanism-based formulation.

Recent longitudinal work supports this approach. Brodbeck et al. (2025) found that the relationship between peer victimisation and later psychopathology was partially mediated by perseverative thinking, threat interpretation bias and emotional reactivity. In other words, the consequences of bullying do not sit only in memory; they can be carried forward through persistent worry, rumination, heightened emotional response and a tendency to interpret social situations as threatening. This has direct clinical relevance. A child who appears oppositional may, in fact, be anticipating attack. A young person who withdraws socially may not simply lack confidence, but may be operating from a learned expectation that social contact is unsafe. Recovery, therefore, requires more than reassurance. It requires intervention at the level of meaning-making, emotional regulation and social prediction.

Recovery as a Multi-level Process

A clinically useful model of recovery from bullying should include four interacting domains: neural, emotional, behavioural and social recovery. These domains are analytically distinct, but in practice they overlap continuously.

Neural recovery refers to the gradual recalibration of stress and social processing systems. The available evidence suggests that victimised young people may show altered activation in regions implicated in social pain, reward, affect and control, alongside heightened sensitivity during acute social exclusion (Ke et al., 2022). From a clinical perspective, this means that recovery often involves helping the young person tolerate social cues without defaulting to alarm, shame or compensatory over-monitoring. The aim is not to claim that therapy simply 'rewires' the brain in a crude sense, but to recognise that repeated safe, regulated and corrective experiences can support adaptive neuroplasticity over time.

Emotional recovery refers to the reduction of fear, shame, humiliation, anger, hopelessness and self-blame. Many bullied children do not merely feel sad; they come to experience themselves as socially defective, permanently vulnerable or fundamentally unlikeable. These appraisals are often sustained by rumination and a biased interpretation of subsequent interactions. Emotional recovery therefore requires both symptom relief and a shift in self-meaning. A child must begin to feel not only calmer, but less contaminated by the bullying experience.

Behavioural recovery refers to the restoration of functioning. This includes sleep, attendance, concentration, participation, social engagement and the capacity to tolerate ordinary developmental demands. It also includes the reduction of defensive or reactive behaviour such as school refusal, avoidance, checking, explosive anger, retaliatory aggression or self-harm. Behavioural improvement is often the most visible marker of progress, but it should not be mistaken for complete recovery. A young person may behave better while remaining deeply dysregulated internally.

Social recovery refers to the rebuilding of trust, belonging and relational safety. Bullying is a social injury, which means recovery cannot be fully understood in intrapsychic terms alone. A child who leaves therapy feeling better, but returns each day to a humiliating peer culture, a dismissive school response or relational isolation is unlikely to recover fully. Social repair requires attention to peer context, family response, school climate and the availability of meaningful support across settings.

Taken together, these domains are consistent with recent work linking peer victimisation with altered social and affective processing, repetitive negative thinking, emotional reactivity and later mental health difficulties (Ke et al., 2022; Brodbeck et al., 2025).

Moving Beyond a Victim-only Model

One of the weaknesses in clinical discussions of bullying is the tendency to imagine a passive victim on one side and an active perpetrator on the other. In reality, a significant subgroup occupies both roles. These bully-victims are often the most distressed and the most clinically complex.

Recent profile research shows that bully-victims report particularly poor psychosocial functioning. In Pivec et al. (2023), bully-victims showed the highest levels of internalising and externalising anger, the lowest levels of anger control, low peer and teacher support, and poor social self-concept. This matters because such presentations are easily misread. A young person who lashes out, intimidates others or appears provocative may still be living with trauma-related shame, rejection sensitivity and persistent dysregulation. Their aggression is not excused by that history, but neither should it be understood outside of it.

The bully-victim profile also appears to carry longer-term risk. Bettencourt et al. (2023) found that high bully-victims were significantly less likely to graduate from high school on time, while pathways involving suspensions and reading attainment helped explain later difficulties. This is a particularly important reminder for clinicians. Bullying involvement can alter not only emotional wellbeing, but also educational trajectory, disciplinary exposure and later social outcomes. A clinically serious recovery model cannot limit itself to internalising symptoms alone, because bullying involvement may also shape educational, behavioural and developmental trajectories (Bettencourt et al., 2023).

Assessing Bullying in Clinical Practice

For clinicians, this complexity has immediate implications for assessment. It is not enough to ask only whether a child has been targeted. One must also explore how the child responds when distressed, whether they retaliate, whether they have become feared or rejected by peers, whether anger is directed inward or outward, and whether aggression has become a maladaptive strategy for managing humiliation or vulnerability. A trauma-informed approach does not mean minimising harm done to others. Rather, it requires recognition that some children present with trauma and aggression at the same time, and that both demand clinical attention.

This is one reason why bullying must be assessed more deliberately in health and mental health settings. Yet, clinicians are often among the first professionals to encounter its consequences, particularly when children present with headaches, abdominal pain, sleep disturbance, anxiety, school avoidance, depressed mood, irritability, concentration problems or suicidal ideation. In primary care, Hutson et al. (2019) found that just over half of paediatric primary care providers reported screening for bullying, and that common interventions included counselling, referral to mental health services and documentation in the clinical record. They also found that stronger attitudes toward screening and higher self-efficacy predicted whether providers actually screened more than knowledge alone. This suggests that missed identification is not simply a problem of information, but also one of clinical confidence and routine practice.

Assessment should therefore begin with the recognition that bullying is often hidden behind more familiar presenting complaints. A child may not arrive at a clinic saying that they are being bullied. Instead, they may present with panic symptoms, self-harm, unexplained somatic complaints, repeated requests not to attend school, or a sudden deterioration in mood, confidence or behaviour. Bullying should be included routinely in psychosocial enquiry when children and adolescents present in this way. Enquiry should also include cyberbullying, because online victimisation can extend humiliation beyond school hours and intensify a sense of inescapability (Hutson et al., 2019).

At the same time, assessment must distinguish bullying from ordinary peer conflict. A clinically useful definition includes repeated aggression, a power imbalance, and actual or likely repetition over time, because a one-off disagreement between equals is not the same as repeated humiliation directed at a child who cannot easily defend themselves (Hutson et al., 2019). Recent measurement work strengthens this point. Strout et al. (2018) developed the Child Adolescent Bullying Scale as a clinically oriented instrument for healthcare settings, designed to reflect the current definition of bullying and support early identification of young people at risk of adverse health outcomes secondary to bullying victimisation. The instrument showed promising screening performance, including good internal consistency, sensitivity of 84 percent, specificity of 65 percent, and an area under the receiver operating characteristic (ROC) curve of 0.74.

No screening tool, however, should replace clinical judgement. The value of a measure such as the Child Adolescent Bullying Scale lies in structuring enquiry and improving early identification, not in reducing a complex developmental and relational experience to a single score. Clinicians still need to establish who is involved, how long the behaviour has been occurring, where it takes place, whether there is a clear or perceived power differential, how the child responds, and whether online victimisation is compounding the harm. This is particularly important in more complex presentations, including bully-victims, where the child may be both harmed by peers and behaving aggressively towards others.

Assessment should also be multi-informant wherever possible. Young people may minimise victimisation because of shame, fear of retaliation or the belief that disclosure will not change anything. Parents may notice school refusal, sleep disruption, physical complaints or a collapse in confidence before the child is able to explain the reason. In the Dutch TRAILS cohort, Kretschmer et al. (2025) found that parent-reported peer victimisation at age 11 was the most stable predictor of later maladjustment, including internalising symptoms, thought problems and somatic complaints, into adolescence and adulthood. Clinically, this supports a formulation process that takes parent observations seriously rather than relying solely on the child's immediate self-report.

A careful bullying assessment therefore does more than identify exposure (Strout et al., 2018; Hutson et al., 2019; Kretschmer et al., 2025). It clarifies pattern, context, meaning and response. It asks not only what happened, but what the child has learned from it, how their social world has changed, and whether their distress is now being maintained by hypervigilance, rumination, shame, avoidance or retaliation. From that point, assessment can move beyond identification and into formulation.

Clinical Priorities at First Presentation

When bullying is disclosed, the first clinical task is not to move immediately into reassurance or treatment planning, but to establish priorities. For some children and adolescents, bullying will be painful, but not acutely dangerous. For others, it may sit alongside escalating self-harm, suicidal ideation, severe school refusal, retaliatory aggression, panic symptoms or ongoing cyberbullying that extends the experience of threat beyond school hours. A careful first presentation therefore requires triage, as well as empathy. Hutson et al. (2019) found that bullying is still not consistently screened in primary care, despite the fact that clinicians often encounter its consequences in the form of low mood, anxiety, somatic complaints, sleep disruption and school-related distress. This underlines the importance of recognising bullying not as a peripheral social issue, but as a potentially significant driver of emotional and behavioural deterioration.

A useful first step is to clarify whether the bullying is current, recent or historical, and whether the young person remains exposed to the same peer group, online environment or social dynamics. Ongoing exposure changes the clinical task. Where the bullying is active and continuing, assessment must include immediate safety, the risk of further victimisation, the possibility of self-harm or suicidal thinking, and the likelihood of retaliation or aggression towards others. Where the bullying has ceased, the emphasis may shift more towards the residual effects, such as rumination, hypervigilance, avoidance, shame or reduced confidence. In both situations, clinicians need to distinguish between the ending of incidents and the ending of impact. Recovery cannot be assumed simply because the observable behaviour has reduced.

At first presentation, it is also important to determine whether the child's distress is primarily internalising, externalising or mixed. Some young people present with tearfulness, panic, stomach aches, nausea, school refusal and social withdrawal. Others present with irritability, anger, defiance, fights or disciplinary problems. As Pivec et al. (2023) show, bully-victims may have particularly poor anger control, low social self-concept and reduced peer and teacher support, making them especially vulnerable to being misread as merely disruptive. This means that early assessment must not stop at the question of whether bullying has occurred. It must also consider how the young person is now coping, how others are responding to them, and whether aggression has become a maladaptive strategy for managing humiliation, fear or social rejection.

The first presentation should therefore establish four broad priorities. The first is immediate risk, including suicidality, self-harm, exposure to ongoing threat or escalating violence. The second is functional deterioration, such as non-attendance, sleep disturbance, panic symptoms, refusal to eat, obsessive checking of phones or messages, or collapse in ordinary daily routines. The third is maintaining mechanisms, including rumination, shame, avoidance, emotional reactivity and biased interpretation of social threat, all of which are supported by the mediation findings reported by Brodbeck et al. (2025). The fourth is support context, including parental awareness, school response, safeguarding action and whether the young person has any safe relational base from which recovery can begin.

In practical terms, this means that the first session or assessment contact should not try to do everything. Its purpose is to clarify whether the presentation requires immediate safeguarding, urgent emotional containment, school liaison, mental health referral or fuller psychological assessment. A young person who is actively suicidal, severely school avoidant or under daily online attack requires a different initial response from one whose bullying exposure has stopped, but who remains stuck in shame, distrust and emotional reactivity. Early clinical work should therefore begin with safety, stabilisation and clear formulation priorities. That approach is consistent with the broader public health position that early identification and coordinated intervention matter if longer-term harm is to be reduced (Dailey et al., 2025).

From Assessment to Formulation

Once bullying has been identified, the next task is not merely to label the child as a victim and offer reassurance. Clinicians need a formulation that explains how the bullying experience is operating in this particular young person. Brodbeck et al. (2025) found that the associations between peer victimisation and later psychopathology were partially mediated by perseverative thinking, threat interpretation bias and emotional reactivity. In practical terms, this means that repeated bullying may leave the child not only distressed, but cognitively and emotionally organised around danger. They may ruminate on past humiliations, interpret ambiguous social cues as hostile and respond with heightened emotional intensity. These mechanisms help explain why the psychological impact of bullying may persist even after the visible incidents have reduced.

A trauma-informed formulation therefore asks several questions. What does the child now expect from other people. How quickly do they detect threat. Do they become flooded by shame, panic or anger. Do they cope by avoiding, masking, appeasing, retaliating or attacking first. Are they trapped in repetitive negative thinking. Have they come to see themselves as weak, unlikeable or permanently unsafe. This approach shifts the clinical focus from what is wrong with the child to what the child has learned to expect in response to repeated social threat. Brodbeck et al. (2025) explicitly argue that such findings support personalised, mechanism-based treatment planning based on adversity profile.

This is particularly important for bully-victims. Pivec et al. (2023) found that bully-victims showed the highest levels of victimisation and bullying involvement, and that profiles involving greater bullying and victimisation were associated with psychosocial adjustment problems. They also reported that victims and bully-victims had the lowest perceived social self-concept, and that lower anger control may increase the risk of further victimisation. This matters clinically because young people who lash out may still be operating from trauma, humiliation and chronic dysregulation, even while harming others.

The bully-victim profile also appears to carry longer-term developmental risk. Bettencourt et al. (2023) identified high-involvement and moderate-involvement bully-victim groups in first grade and found that, compared with low or no involvement peers, high bully-victims were less likely to graduate high school on time, while moderate bully-victims were more likely to have later criminal justice involvement. Reading attainment and school suspensions partly explained these pathways, suggesting that the consequences of bullying involvement are not limited to emotional distress alone, but may extend into educational and behavioural trajectories.

Bullying participation also cannot always be reduced to a simple bully or victim dichotomy. Pivec et al. (2023) identified five subgroups: uninvolved students, self-reported uninvolved students, bullies, victims, and bully-victims. They showed that the different profiles varied across psychosocial characteristics such as peer and teacher support, anger expression and social self-concept. This supports a more nuanced clinical view in which some young people move between positions of vulnerability, retaliation and social performance rather than occupying one fixed role.

This complexity becomes clearer when translated into clinical practice. A formulation is only useful if it helps the clinician decide what to notice, what to ask next, and what kind of intervention is likely to be most helpful. In bullying-related presentations, the same underlying experience of repeated humiliation, exclusion or fear may produce very different outward patterns. One child may become angry, provocative and retaliatory. Another may become withdrawn, self-critical and physically unwell. Both may be responding to chronic social threat, but the pathway through which that threat is processed, expressed and maintained can differ substantially. As Brodbeck et al. (2025) argue, adversity-related psychopathology is better understood through mediating mechanisms such as perseverative thinking, threat interpretation bias and emotional reactivity than through simple exposure categories alone.

The following case illustrations are composites intended to reflect common clinical patterns; all names and identifying details have been changed to preserve confidentiality.

Box 7.1 Clinical Case Illustration: Jake

Jake is 13 and is referred after striking another pupil at school. Staff describe him as angry, oppositional and increasingly disruptive. At first glance, he appears to fit a conduct-focused profile. His mother, however, reports that over the previous six months he has become reluctant to attend school, complains of stomach aches on Sunday evenings, and checks social media repeatedly late at night. He insists that he does not care what others think, yet becomes visibly tense when discussing one particular friendship group.

A more detailed assessment reveals repeated victimisation by peers who mock his appearance, exclude him from group activities, and provoke him online before denying responsibility when adults intervene. Jake has begun retaliating physically and verbally. He reports constant thoughts about what others are saying about him, replays humiliating incidents in his mind, and assumes that laughter nearby is directed at him. He is ashamed of feeling hurt and vulnerable, so he presents anger rather than fear. In formulation terms, Jake's difficulties are consistent with the mechanisms described by Brodbeck et al. (2025), particularly threat interpretation bias, perseverative thinking and heightened emotional reactivity. His presentation also reflects the bully-victim profile described by Pivec et al. (2023), in which victimisation, aggression, low anger control and poor social self-concept may co-exist.

Jake's case illustrates why a trauma-informed formulation must not collapse into a victim-only model. His aggression requires response, but it should not be understood only as wilful misconduct. The available evidence suggests that bully-victims may be among the most dysregulated young people, with elevated anger problems, reduced anger control, and poor peer and teacher support (Pivec et al., 2023). Longer-term research also indicates that more highly involved bully-victims are at risk of later educational and behavioural difficulties, including the reduced likelihood of graduating on time and greater involvement with the criminal justice system, with suspensions and academic underachievement contributing to these pathways (Bettencourt et al., 2023). In Jake's case, a purely punitive response to fighting would miss the trauma-related processes maintaining his distress, while a purely supportive response that ignored the harm he is doing to others would be equally incomplete.

Box 7.2 Clinical Case Illustration: Maya

Maya is 12 and presents in primary care with headaches, poor sleep, nausea before school and increasing tearfulness. Initial physical investigations are unremarkable. She is quiet in consultation and says little unless prompted directly. Her mother reports that Maya used to enjoy school, but now asks to stay home, has stopped attending clubs, and spends long periods alone in her bedroom.

Gentle questioning reveals that Maya has become the target of repeated exclusion and hostility within friendship groups and online spaces. Other girls remove her from group chats, post photographs without her, and imply that she is unlikeable, then deny that anything is wrong when confronted. Maya says she feels foolish for being upset and has begun to believe that nobody would want to spend time with her anyway. She repeatedly rereads messages after school, searching for signs that people dislike her, and has started interpreting even neutral looks from classmates as evidence that she is being judged.

Maya's presentation is quieter than Jake's, but no less serious. Her difficulties are primarily internalising, with shame, social threat sensitivity, avoidance, negative self-appraisal, disturbed sleep and repetitive negative thinking all now maintaining distress. This pattern is also consistent with the mechanism-based account offered by Brodbeck et al. (2025), in which peer victimisation contributes to later psychopathology partly through perseverative thinking and biased threat interpretation. Maya has not become aggressive towards others, but she has nonetheless reorganised her social world around danger, rejection and self-doubt.

Taken together, Jake and Maya illustrate an important clinical point. Bullying does not produce one standard presentation. The same underlying experience of repeated interpersonal harm may lead one young person towards retaliatory aggression and another towards withdrawal, rumination and physical symptoms. This is why formulation must sit at the centre of recovery planning. Without formulation, intervention risks becoming generic, reactive or overly focused on the most visible symptom.

From Formulation to Intervention

Once the clinician has established how bullying is being processed and maintained in the individual child, intervention can be more precisely targeted. The aim is not simply to reduce immediate distress, but to interrupt the mechanisms through which the bullying experience continues to shape mood, behaviour, relationships and self-perception. This means that intervention should address both symptoms and maintaining processes, including rumination, hypervigilance, shame, emotional dysregulation, avoidance and retaliatory behaviour where present.

For children whose presentations include intrusive distress, fear, avoidance, hyperarousal and persistent dysregulation, trauma-focused approaches are highly relevant. Thielemann et al. (2022) found that trauma-focused cognitive behavioural therapy was associated with substantial pre- to post-treatment improvement in post-traumatic stress symptoms and favourable effects relative to control conditions, with benefits also observed for depressive, anxiety and grief symptoms. They conclude that TF-CBT is an effective intervention for paediatric trauma symptoms and supports international guidance recommending it as a first-line treatment. In bullying-related cases, this evidence is particularly useful because it supports a structured intervention that does more than offer reassurance. It provides a framework for psychoeducation, relaxation, affect modulation, cognitive coping, trauma narrative work where appropriate, caregiver involvement and safety planning.

For a young person such as Jake, intervention is likely to require explicit work on anger regulation, the hostile interpretation of social cues, shame and retaliatory patterns, alongside active school involvement to reduce ongoing victimisation and limit the reinforcement of aggression. For a young person such as Maya, the therapeutic focus may be more strongly centred on self-blame, rumination, avoidance, social confidence and the rebuilding of emotional safety. In both cases, however, treatment should not be confined to the therapy room. Dailey et al. (2025) emphasise the importance of screening and early identification, family and community involvement, attention to mental health and wellbeing, multi-component school-based approaches, and coordinated intervention across systems. Recovery is therefore most likely when the child experiences consistency across clinical care, family response and school practice.

The role of family support should also be framed carefully. Supportive relationships matter, but they are not an automatic buffer against harm. Martínez et al. (2024) found that greater peer victimisation predicted increases in depressive, separation anxiety, and ADHD symptoms over time. Although parental warmth was associated with lower depressive symptoms, it did not consistently moderate the association between victimisation and all mental health outcomes. Prosocial school environments appeared to buffer depressive symptoms, but they were not uniformly protective across all presentations. This is an important reminder that resilience should not be romanticised. Warmth, support and belonging matter deeply, but some children require more intensive and sustained intervention to undo the effects of repeated social threat.

The question then becomes not whether intervention is needed, but which targets should come first.

Deciding between Intervention Priorities

Once bullying has been identified and the initial priorities are clear, the clinician must decide what to address first. This is where formulation becomes indispensable. Two children may both have been repeatedly bullied, yet one may be dominated by panic, intrusive imagery and avoidance, while another may be dominated by shame, anger, rumination and retaliatory behaviour. To apply the same intervention sequence to both would be clinically imprecise. As Brodbeck et al. (2025) suggest, repeated adversity may contribute to later psychopathology through mechanisms such as perseverative thinking, threat interpretation bias and emotional reactivity. These mechanisms provide a useful basis for deciding treatment priorities.

For some young people, the first priority will be stabilisation and emotional regulation. This is especially important where the child is highly distressed, sleep deprived, panicky, emotionally flooded, or engaging in self-harm or repeated crisis behaviours. In such cases, immediate trauma processing or detailed cognitive work may be premature. The child may first need help in recognising bodily activation, identifying escalation cues, practising calming strategies and reducing exposure to ongoing triggers, particularly online triggers. Where the young person cannot yet tolerate discussion of the bullying without becoming overwhelmed, regulation work is not a delay to treatment, but the beginning of it.

For others, the first priority will be cognitive and meaning-based work. Some children remain distressed, not because the incidents are ongoing, but because they continue to interpret themselves and other people through the lens of humiliation. They expect rejection, assume mockery and scan relentlessly for signs that they are unlikeable or unsafe. In these cases, treatment may need to focus earlier on self-blame, distorted threat interpretation and repetitive negative thinking. This is particularly relevant in quieter, more internalising presentations, where distress may otherwise be mistaken for shyness, oversensitivity or ordinary adolescent insecurity. Maya-like presentations often require careful work on shame, social prediction and avoidance before confidence can begin to recover.

A different set of priorities emerges in bully-victim presentations. Here, treatment may need to address trauma and aggression at the same time. Jake-like presentations are clinically challenging because the young person is both harmed and harming. Work focused only on their pain may fail to address the damage they are causing to others, while work focused only on behaviour may miss the shame, humiliation and hypervigilance driving their reactivity. Pivec et al. (2023) and Bettencourt et al. (2023) together support the view that children involved in both victimisation and perpetration may follow particularly adverse developmental pathways, with difficulties extending into school exclusion, poorer educational progress and later behavioural problems. For these young people, early priorities may include anger regulation, work on hostile attribution, reduction of retaliatory responses and explicit planning for safer peer encounters, alongside acknowledgment of their own victimisation history.

Another key decision concerns the role of caregivers. In some cases, parental understanding and emotional availability are central to recovery. In others, parents may be unaware of the scale of the problem, unsure how to respond, or unintentionally increasing distress through repeated questioning, anger towards the school or pressure on the child to 'stand up for themselves'. Thielemann et al. (2022) describe TF-CBT as involving caregiver participation in psychoeducation, affect regulation, cognitive coping, trauma processing and safety enhancement. This is highly relevant in bullying-related cases. Caregivers often need help understanding that the child's presentation may reflect chronic social threat rather than weakness, attention-seeking or bad behaviour. Without that understanding, home may become another setting in which the child feels blamed or misunderstood.

The final major intervention priority is school liaison and environmental change. No therapy can work effectively if the child continues to return to an unchanged environment of humiliation, exclusion or threat. This does not mean that clinicians should take over the school's role, but it does mean that recovery planning should include, with appropriate consent, communication about safety, attendance, support, friendship arrangements, online bullying and reintegration. Dailey et al. (2025) emphasise that responses to bullying are strongest when healthcare, public health, families and schools work in a coordinated way rather than in parallel. In practice, clinicians need to ask not only what the young person feels, but what will have to change in their environment for those feelings to become less reasonable.

Intervention and Recovery Planning

Intervention should be matched to formulation. Not every bullied child requires the same treatment, and not every distressed presentation after bullying is best conceptualised as post-traumatic stress. However, where symptoms include intrusive distress, avoidance, hyperarousal, fear, shame and persistent dysregulation, trauma-focused approaches are highly relevant. Thielemann et al. (2022) found that TF-CBT produced large pre- to post-treatment improvements in post-traumatic stress symptoms and favourable results relative to control conditions, with benefits also seen for depressive, anxiety and grief symptoms. They conclude that TF-CBT is an effective treatment for paediatric post-traumatic stress symptoms, and support international guidance recommending it as a first-line treatment.

For bullying-related presentations, this evidence suggests several principles. First, treatment should address both symptoms and mechanisms. It is not enough to reduce immediate distress if the young person's thinking remains dominated by rumination, humiliation and threat expectation. Second, caregiver involvement matters. Thielemann et al. (2022) describe TF-CBT as including psychoeducation and parenting skills, relaxation, affective modulation, cognitive coping, trauma narrative work, *in vivo* exposure where appropriate, conjoint parent–child sessions, and enhancing safety and development, with caregiver participation treated as integral rather than optional.

Support outside therapy also matters, but the evidence is more nuanced than simple resilience language implies. Martínez et al. (2024) found that higher exposure to peer victimisation was associated with increases in depressive, separation anxiety and ADHD symptoms over time. Parental warmth was associated with decreases in depressive symptoms, but did not robustly buffer the link between peer victimisation and all mental health outcomes. Prosocial school environments buffered the link with depressive symptoms, but amplified associations with separation anxiety and ADHD symptoms. Their conclusion was that parental warmth and prosocial school environments may not be enough to counter the negative consequences of peer victimisation across all outcomes.

This is why recovery planning should be multi-systemic. A child cannot recover fully if therapy and home are supportive, but the school context remains unsafe or humiliating. Dailey et al. (2025) identified six key themes in healthcare and public health interventions: screening and early identification, family and community involvement, attention to mental health and wellbeing, multi-component school-based work, cognitive-behavioural and solution-focused interventions, and online and digital interventions. They argue that healthcare and public health professionals are well placed to contribute to early identification, prevention and resilience-building, but that stronger cross-sector collaboration remains necessary.

The clinician's role, therefore, is not simply to reduce symptoms in isolation, but to help rebuild a developmental pathway. For some children that will mean reducing panic, rumination and school refusal. For others it will mean helping them regulate anger, step out of retaliatory patterns and develop safer ways of responding to humiliation. Across presentations, recovery involves more than symptom suppression. It involves restoring a workable sense of safety in self, in relationships and in the future. The neurobiological literature also supports this cautious view, suggesting associations between peer victimisation and the altered processing of social reward, social exclusion and affect, rather than a simplistic claim of fixed damage (Ke et al., 2022).

Monitoring Recovery in Practice

Recovery from bullying should be monitored with the same seriousness as its initial assessment. A common clinical mistake is to assume that improvement can be judged simply by asking whether the bullying has stopped or whether the child feels 'better'. While both questions matter, they are too limited to capture the wider process of recovery described in this chapter. A child may report fewer incidents, but remain frightened, self-critical, sleepless or socially avoidant. Another may appear calmer, but may still be checking messages obsessively, missing school or becoming enraged in response to minor peer stress. Monitoring therefore needs to track not only symptom reduction, but also change in functioning, relationships, self-perception and regulation.

A useful recovery review includes several domains. The first is emotional change, including reductions in anxiety, panic, shame, sadness, irritability and emotional flooding. The second is cognitive change, such as less rumination, fewer threat-based interpretations of ambiguous social situations and reduced preoccupation with humiliation or rejection. These domains are especially important in light of Brodbeck et al. (2025), whose work suggests that perseverative thinking, threat interpretation bias and emotional reactivity are not incidental features of bullying recovery, but central mechanisms through which distress may persist. If these processes remain unchanged, apparent surface improvement may be fragile.

The third domain is behavioural and functional change. This includes attendance, punctuality, concentration, sleep, appetite, school participation, use of social media, frequency of somatic complaints and willingness to resume ordinary activities such as clubs, friendships or family outings. In younger people, recovery may also be visible in reduced clinginess, fewer morning meltdowns, or greater willingness to separate from parents. In bully-victim presentations, behavioural monitoring should include incidents of retaliation, verbal aggression, disciplinary episodes or online conflict, because improved emotional insight does not automatically translate into safer behaviour.

The fourth domain is relational and environmental change. Recovery is less likely to hold if the child remains isolated, unsupported or exposed to subtle forms of ongoing exclusion. Martínez et al. (2024) show that support matters, but not in a simplistic or uniform way. Parental warmth was associated with lower depressive symptoms, but did not consistently buffer all the consequences of peer victimisation, while prosocial school environments were protective for some outcomes, but not all. This means that clinicians should monitor the quality, consistency and usefulness of support, rather than merely noting that support exists in principle. A child may have a caring parent and still feel socially unsafe. Another may have friends and still be trapped in online hostility.

In practice, monitoring recovery can be assisted by structured reviews at agreed intervals. Clinicians may wish to revisit specific goals such as school attendance, reduced phone checking, fewer somatic complaints, improved sleep, reduction in self-harm urges or greater confidence in peer situations. Where a screening tool has been used at assessment, it may also help track change over time, although tools should always sit alongside clinical judgement rather than replace it. The broader aim is to ensure that recovery is being understood as a process of re-engagement with life, not only as a reduction in distress scores.

Barriers to Recovery

Even when bullying is identified and support is offered, recovery is not always straightforward. One reason is that the barriers to recovery are often social as much as psychological. A child may begin to make sense of their experience in therapy, yet continue to return each day to a peer environment that remains hostile, dismissive or subtly excluding. In these circumstances, recovery work risks being undermined by ongoing exposure. Children and adolescents are especially vulnerable to this because their social worlds are not easily escaped. Unlike adults, they often cannot choose a new workplace, friendship network or daily environment. Their recovery remains tied to settings they do not control.

A second barrier is misrecognition by adults. Bullying is still too easily minimised as ordinary peer conflict, friendship drama or part of growing up. Where schools respond defensively, families may feel unheard and children may conclude that disclosure is futile. Hutson et al. (2019) found that bullying is not consistently screened, even in paediatric primary care, which suggests that some young people may reach services only after distress has already become entrenched. In bully-victim presentations, the risk of misrecognition is even greater. A child who has started lashing out may be treated purely as a behavioural problem, with little curiosity about humiliation, fear or rejection. In such cases, the system may respond to the child's adaptation rather than to the injury that gave rise to it.

A third barrier is shame. Shame is one of the most corrosive features of bullying-related distress because it inhibits disclosure, distorts interpretation and isolates the child from help. Young people may feel embarrassed that they were targeted, ashamed that they did not defend themselves, or ashamed that they care so much about what others think. Bully-victims may feel additional shame about their own aggression. Shame also reinforces silence. A child who expects disbelief or ridicule may say very little in clinical encounters, particularly early on. This is one reason why multi-informant assessment is so important, and why parent reports, school observations and careful behavioural enquiry may reveal more than direct self-labelling alone.

A fourth barrier is the persistence of digital exposure. Cyberbullying can make victimisation feel continuous, portable and inescapable. It extends peer surveillance into evenings, weekends and private spaces, increasing the likelihood of sleep disturbance, obsessive checking, anticipatory anxiety and re-exposure to humiliating material. Even where school-based incidents have reduced, the emotional system may remain activated by group chats, photographs, comments or fears about what is being said online. For some young people, the phone becomes both a source of threat and an object they cannot stop monitoring. This can significantly slow recovery unless clinicians ask directly about digital behaviour and help families think about boundaries, evidence capture, reporting and safe use.

Finally, recovery may be obstructed by disciplinary pathways that deepen exclusion rather than restore safety. Bettencourt et al. (2023) found that suspensions partly explained the association between bully-victim involvement and later adverse outcomes. That does not mean that schools should avoid consequences for harmful behaviour. It means that professionals need to recognise when repeated punitive responses are pushing a dysregulated child further away from support, education and repair. For some bully-victims, exclusion from school may compound shame, reduce supervision and intensify identification with anger or rejection. A trauma-informed response should therefore ask not only what sanction is appropriate, but what consequence is most likely to interrupt the harmful developmental pathway.

Taken together, these barriers help explain why recovery is often uneven (Hutson et al., 2019; Bettencourt et al., 2023; Martínez et al., 2024). Progress may occur in one domain, while another remains stuck. A child may sleep better but still refuse school, feel calmer but remain socially isolated, or stop self-harming while continuing to expect rejection from others. Recognising these barriers is clinically important because it prevents simplistic judgements about resistance, non-compliance or treatment failure. Recovery from bullying is not blocked only by what is happening inside the child. It is also shaped by what continues around them, and by how well the adults in their world respond.

Long-term Outcomes and Developmental Sequelae

The need for sustained, formulation-driven intervention becomes even clearer when longer-term outcomes are considered (Brimblecombe et al., 2018; Bettencourt et al., 2023; Kretschmer et al., 2025). Bullying is not only associated with immediate emotional distress or short-term disruption in school functioning. For some young people, its effects extend into later adolescence and adulthood, shaping educational progress, employment, wealth, mental health, service use and broader life chances. This does not mean that all bullied children will experience chronic impairment, nor that recovery is impossible. It does mean, however, that clinicians should avoid treating bullying as a transient developmental difficulty with no enduring consequences. Recent longitudinal evidence suggests that the developmental footprint of bullying can remain visible long after the original incidents have ceased.

One of the clearest recent demonstrations of this comes from Brimblecombe et al. (2018), who examined the economic impact of childhood bullying victimisation at age 50 using the 1958 British birth cohort. They found substantial and durable consequences across both individual and societal domains. Men and women who had been bullied in childhood were less likely to be in employment and had accumulated less wealth, including having lower levels of home ownership and savings than those who had not been bullied. For women, frequent bullying in childhood was associated with lower net weekly earnings from paid employment, while frequent bullying was also linked to higher health service costs for mental health conditions among women and higher employment-related societal costs among men. Importantly, the authors concluded that the consequences of childhood bullying were not only long-lasting, but pervasive, underlining the need for support not only during childhood, but in the decades that follow.

Recent work on bully-victims adds further precision to this picture. Bettencourt et al. (2023) showed that early bully-victim involvement was associated with later educational and behavioural difficulties in early adulthood. High-involvement bully-victims were significantly less likely to graduate from high school on time, while moderate-involvement bully-victims were more likely to become involved with the criminal justice system. The study also found that sixth-grade reading attainment and school suspensions partially explained these pathways. This is an important finding for health and mental health professionals because it shows that bullying involvement may shape adult outcomes not only through later psychiatric symptoms, but through school exclusion, academic disruption and disciplinary escalation. In other words, the aftermath of bullying may become embedded in the young person's developmental pathway, affecting how they move through education and into adult life.

The persistence of maladjustment into adulthood is also illustrated by Kretschmer et al. (2025), using the Dutch TRAILS cohort from age 11 to 29. In that study, parent-reported peer victimisation in early adolescence was the most stable predictor of later maladjustment, including internalising symptoms, thought problems and somatic complaints. Teacher-reported victimisation also predicted later maladjustment, but more weakly, while self and peer reports did not remain stable predictors once all reporters were considered together. This finding matters clinically for two reasons. First, it reinforces the need to take parent observations seriously when young people present with changes in mood, withdrawal, fatigue, headaches, sleep problems or unusual thought content. Second, it demonstrates that the consequences of peer victimisation may remain visible well into adulthood, even when baseline maladjustment and social background factors are taken into account.

This has an important implication for the concept of recovery. Recovery cannot be defined narrowly as the cessation of bullying incidents, or even as the reduction of overt symptoms alone (Brimblecombe et al., 2018; Bettencourt et al., 2023; Kretschmer et al., 2025). A child may no longer be actively targeted, and yet remain socially hypervigilant, ashamed, avoidant or developmentally derailed. Equally, a young person may appear to have 'moved on', while still carrying the educational and relational consequences of earlier peer victimisation. Long-term outcome research therefore strengthens the argument that recovery should be understood as a broader developmental process involving repair of self-worth, trust, regulation, participation and opportunity.

Implications for Health and Mental Health Professionals

For health and mental health professionals, the practical message is clear. If bullying can shape later functioning across mental health, education, employment and social outcomes, then assessment and intervention must be correspondingly broad. It is not enough to ask whether bullying is happening now. Clinicians also need to consider what has already been altered by the experience. Has the child become avoidant of school? Has concentration deteriorated? Has suspension or conflict with peers begun to accumulate? Are there somatic complaints that signal chronic distress? Has the young person become socially withdrawn, persistently angry or deeply self-critical? These questions help clinicians move beyond event-based assessment towards developmental formulation (Brimblecombe et al., 2018; Bettencourt et al., 2023; Kretschmer et al., 2025).

This is also where cross-sector working becomes essential. Dailey et al. (2025) argue that healthcare and public health professionals are uniquely positioned to contribute to early identification, prevention and resilience-building, but that their roles are still not consistently integrated into bullying prevention frameworks. Their review identified six key themes in relevant interventions: screening and early identification, family and community involvement, attention to mental health and wellbeing, multi-component school-based interventions, cognitive–behavioural and solution-focused approaches, and online or digital interventions. The significance of this for Chapter 7 is that it supports a model in which health professionals do more than treat the aftermath in isolation. They can help identify bullying earlier, coordinate care more effectively, and contribute to a more joined-up response across clinical, school, family and community contexts.

For clinicians, this means that recovery planning should remain formulation-led and individually tailored. Children such as Maya may need help with rumination, self-blame and re-entry into social participation, while children such as Jake may need work that explicitly addresses shame, anger, retaliatory responding and school exclusion risk. In both cases, early intervention is likely to matter, because the longer bullying-related difficulties are left to harden into entrenched patterns of avoidance, dysregulation or disciplinary failure, the more likely they are to affect later developmental outcomes. That does not justify alarmism, but it does justify urgency (Bettencourt et al., 2023; Dailey et al., 2025).

Conclusion

Bullying recovery is best understood not as a return to the person the child was before harm occurred, but as a process of rebuilding developmental possibility. Repeated peer victimisation can alter how a young person thinks, feels, behaves, relates to others, and moves through key educational and social transitions. For some, the consequences remain largely internal, taking the form of anxiety, shame, rumination and somatic distress. For others, they become behavioural and relational, expressed through anger, school disruption, retaliation or disengagement. For bully-victims in particular, the developmental picture may be especially complex, as trauma, aggression and poor social support become intertwined.

The evidence reviewed in this chapter suggests that these outcomes are not merely short term. They can persist into adulthood, affecting mental health, educational attainment, criminal justice involvement, employment, wealth and health service use (Brimblecombe et al., 2018; Bettencourt et al., 2023; Kretschmer et al., 2025). Yet, the same evidence also points towards a constructive clinical response. When health and mental health professionals assess bullying deliberately, use multi-informant and mechanism-based formulations, involve families and schools, and intervene early and collaboratively, they are not simply reducing symptoms. They are helping to interrupt the developmental pathways through which bullying can become embedded.

Ultimately, to work effectively with children and adolescents affected by bullying is to take their social injuries seriously. It is to recognise that humiliation, exclusion and chronic peer threat are not trivial rites of passage, but experiences capable of shaping the course of development. The task for professionals is therefore not only to ask whether the bullying has stopped, but whether safety, trust, self-worth and participation have begun to return. That is the real work of recovery (Ke et al., 2022; Dailey et al., 2025).

Key Takeaways

- Recovery from bullying should be understood as neural, emotional, behavioural and social repair
- Peer victimisation can shape threat sensitivity, rumination, emotional reactivity and later functioning
- Bully-victims are often among the most clinically complex young people and may present with both trauma and aggression
- Bullying assessment should be deliberate, multi-informant and attentive to both victimisation and perpetration
- Formulation is essential because bullying does not produce one standard presentation
- Intervention should address symptoms and maintaining mechanisms, including shame, hypervigilance, rumination, avoidance and retaliatory responding
- Recovery is more likely when support is coordinated across clinical care, family response and school practice
- The consequences of bullying may extend well beyond childhood, affecting education, psychosocial functioning and adult outcomes

References

Bettencourt, A.F., Clary, L.K., Ialongo, N. and Musci, R.J. (2023) 'Long-term consequences of bullying involvement in first grade', *Journal of School Psychology*, 97, pp. 63–76. https://doi.org/10.1016/j.jsp.2023.01.004.

Brimblecombe, N., Evans-Lacko, S., Knapp, M., King, D., Takizawa, R., Maughan, B. and Arseneault, L. (2018) 'Long term economic impact associated with childhood bullying victimisation', *Social Science & Medicine*, 208, pp. 134–141. https://doi.org/10.1016/j.socscimed.2018.05.014.

Brodbeck, J., Jacinto, S., Stallmann, L., Vetsch, N., Marmet, S. and Neufeld, S.A. (2025) 'Perseverative thinking, threat interpretation bias, and emotional reactivity as mediators between adverse childhood experience domains and psychopathology: A longitudinal mediation study in a cohort of Swiss emerging adults', *International*

Journal of Clinical and Health Psychology, [online] 25(4), p. 100654. doi:10.1016/j.ijchp.2025.100654.

Dailey, S.F., Roche, R.R. and Sharkey, M.C. (2025) 'Addressing bullying and cyberbullying in public health: A systematic review of interventions for healthcare and public health professionals', *International Journal of Environmental Research and Public Health*, [online] 22(11), p. 1682. doi:10.3390/ijerph22111682.

Hutson, E., Melnyk, B., Hensley, V. and Sinnott, L.T. (2019) 'Childhood bullying: Screening and intervening practices of pediatric primary care providers', *Journal of Pediatric Health Care*, [online] 33(6), pp. e39–e45. https://doi.org/10.1016/j.pedhc.2019.07.003.

Ke, T., De Simoni, S., Barker, E. and Smith, P. (2022) 'The association between peer-victimisation and structural and functional brain outcomes: A systematic review', *JCPP Advances*, [online] 2, p. e12081. doi:10.1002/jcv2.12081.

Kretschmer, T., Van der Ploeg, R. and Kaufman, T. (2025) 'Peer victimization in early adolescence and maladjustment in adulthood', *European Child & Adolescent Psychiatry*, 34(3), pp. 1011–1024. https://doi.org/10.1007/s00787-024-02532-5.

Martínez, M., Damme, K.S., Vargas, T., Yang, B., Rompilla, D.J., Stephens, J., Qu, Y., Mittal, V.A. and Haase, C.M. (2024) 'Longitudinal study of peer victimization, social support, and mental health during early adolescence', *Psychological Medicine*, 54(9), pp. 1940–1955. https://doi.org/10.1017/S0033291724000035.

Pivec, T., Horvat, M. and Košir, K. (2023) 'Psychosocial characteristics of bullying participants: A person-oriented approach combining self- and peer-report measures', *Children and Youth Services Review*, [online] 144, p. 106720. doi:10.1016/j.childyouth.2022.106720.

Strout, T.D., Vessey, J.A., DiFazio, R.L. and Ludlow, L.H. (2018) 'The Child Adolescent Bullying Scale (CABS): Psychometric evaluation of a new measure', *Research in Nursing & Health*, 41(3), pp. 252–264. https://doi.org/10.1002/nur.21871.

Thielemann, J.F.B., Kasparik, B., König, J., Unterhitzenberger, J. and Rosner, R. (2022) 'A systematic review and meta-analysis of trauma-focused cognitive behavioral therapy for children and adolescents', *Child Abuse & Neglect*, [online] 134, p. 105899. doi:10.1016/j.chiabu.2022.105899.

Chapter 8

Taking Action

Advice for Policymakers and Professionals

Abstract

Bullying is not a minor disciplinary problem, but a public health, educational, safeguarding and equity issue with consequences for wellbeing, learning, belonging and longer-term development. This chapter translates the evidence reviewed throughout the book into practical recommendations for policymakers, educators and health professionals. Drawing on recent international and school-based evidence, it argues that effective responses must move beyond standalone policies and awareness campaigns towards coordinated, whole-system approaches that integrate school culture, family engagement, mental health support, inclusion and digital safety. The chapter highlights the importance of implementation quality, staff preparedness, reporting confidence and school belonging, alongside clearer accountability and stronger support for children with special educational needs and disabilities. It also argues that success should be judged not only by reductions in reported bullying, but by whether children feel safe, seek help, trust adults and remain connected to school. Sustained, evidence-informed and inclusive action is essential if bullying prevention is to produce meaningful and lasting change.

In This Chapter

- Why bullying requires a systems response
- What policymakers should do
- What education systems and schools should do
- Inclusion, special educational needs and disability-responsive practice
- What health and mental health professionals should do
- Cyberbullying and digital harm
- Implementation, evaluation and accountability
- Conclusion and key takeaways

Bullying is not a minor part of growing up, nor is it a routine pastoral issue that can be managed through isolated sanctions or brief awareness campaigns. It

DOI: 10.4324/9781003771777-12

is a serious threat to emotional wellbeing, educational participation, social development and longer-term mental health. For many children and young people, the effects of bullying extend beyond immediate incidents. They shape confidence, belonging, trust in others, school attendance and willingness to seek help. When bullying is persistent, ignored or poorly handled, its impact can become embedded in the wider developmental experience of childhood and adolescence.

Recent international evidence reinforces the scale and urgency of the problem. The WHO Health Behaviour in School-aged Children report, drawing on data from 44 countries and regions, found that bullying and cyberbullying remain significant concerns across adolescence, and called for stronger action across schools, families and communities (WHO Regional Office for Europe, 2024). This matters because it places bullying firmly beyond the category of a local or isolated school issue. It is a cross-national challenge that affects educational equity, public health, child safety and social inclusion.

The research base also shows that effective action is rarely simple. Whole-school interventions remain important, but their impact is often shaped by implementation quality, staff confidence, school climate and the extent to which prevention is embedded in everyday systems rather than treated as an additional task (Lekamge et al., 2025). Healthcare and public health professionals are also frequently under-integrated into anti-bullying work, despite being well placed to identify distress, support families and strengthen recovery pathways (Dailey et al., 2025). This suggests that bullying should be approached not as a single behavioural problem, but as a systems issue requiring coordinated responses across education, health, safeguarding, family life and digital environments.

This chapter therefore moves from evidence to action. It considers what policymakers, education professionals, and health and mental health practitioners should do to reduce bullying, respond more effectively when it occurs, and support children and young people in recovery. It also addresses the importance of inclusion, especially for pupils with special educational needs and disabilities, and argues that accountability should extend beyond written policies and incident counts to include belonging, safety, help-seeking and the quality of adult response. In doing so, the chapter makes the case that meaningful anti-bullying action must be evidence-informed, inclusive and sustained over time.

Why Bullying Requires a Systems Response

Bullying is often discussed as though it were primarily a matter of individual behaviour. In practice, however, it is shaped by a much wider set of conditions, including school climate, peer norms, consistency of adult response, family relationships, access to support, and the online environments in which children now spend much of their social lives. This means that anti-bullying work cannot succeed through isolated lessons, reactive sanctions or written policies alone. A narrow behavioural model may capture the incident itself, but it does not adequately address the culture, context and systems that allow bullying to persist.

Recent evidence supports this broader view. A systematic review and meta-analysis of whole-school interventions found significant reductions in cyberbullying and cyber aggression, but also concluded that many mixed or non-significant findings were likely linked to weaknesses in implementation and in how the wider Health Promoting Schools framework was translated into practice (Lekamge et al., 2025). This is an important message for policymakers and practitioners alike. It suggests that the challenge is not simply whether an intervention exists, but whether it is properly embedded, supported, adapted and sustained.

A systems approach is also necessary because bullying is closely linked to wider educational experiences such as belonging, fairness and trust in adults. Positive teacher–student relationships have been associated with improved wellbeing, attendance, engagement, inclusion and sense of school belonging, all of which are relevant to bullying prevention and recovery (Nix et al., 2022). Similarly, research on school safety has shown that feeling safe is shaped not only by bullying victimisation itself, but by the overall climate of the school, including consistent rules, positive relationships and a strong sense of belonging (Williams et al., 2018). These findings indicate that successful anti-bullying work depends on whether schools are experienced as relationally safe environments, not merely whether they can evidence a policy document.

The issue of help-seeking further strengthens the systems argument. Bullied children and adolescents do not always disclose to professionals what is happening. Grüne and Willems (2024) found that, although many bullied adolescents sought help, most relied on informal sources such as family and friends, with far fewer using formal support routes. This matters because it means that schools and services cannot assume that pupils will naturally disclose to staff. If reporting pathways are unclear, adults are poorly prepared, or trust is low, harm may remain hidden. Gizzarelli et al. (2023) further found that staff responses to reports of bullying can be inconsistent, and in some cases absent altogether, while staff preparedness and training were associated with more constructive responses. A systems response is therefore required not only to prevent bullying, but also to ensure that when children seek help, adults are ready to respond effectively.

Taken together, this evidence suggests that bullying should be addressed through a public health, educational and safeguarding lens. It requires coordinated work across policy, school culture, family involvement, health services and digital safety. It also requires a shift in how success is judged. Reducing reported incidents matters, but so too does belonging, perceived safety, attendance, reporting confidence and the credibility of adult response.

Without attention to these wider conditions, anti-bullying work risks becoming procedural rather than protective.

What Policymakers Should Do

If bullying is to be addressed seriously, policymakers must move beyond the assumption that it is simply a matter for individual schools or classroom teachers. The evidence now points towards a broader systems problem that requires coordinated action across education, health, safeguarding and digital policy. Recent international data from the WHO Health Behaviour in School-aged Children survey, covering 44 countries and regions, show that peer violence and bullying remain significant concerns across adolescence, with over one in ten young people reporting repeated bullying at school and higher levels of cyberbullying exposure. The report concludes that further investment is needed in family, school and community-based interventions, and identifies cyberbullying as an urgent policy priority (WHO Regional Office for Europe, 2024).

Within England, this systems response is already distributed across a number of overlapping policy and legal frameworks rather than contained in a single anti-bullying statute.

Within England, anti-bullying policy sits across behaviour, safeguarding, equality, special educational needs and disabilities, the curriculum and online safety frameworks. Key foundations include section 89 of the Education and Inspections Act 2006 (Great Britain, 2006), the Department for Education's *Preventing and Tackling Bullying* guidance (Department for Education, 2017), *Behaviour in Schools, Keeping Children Safe in Education* (Department for Education, 2025a), the Equality Act 2010 (Great Britain, 2010), the Children and Families Act 2014 (Great Britain, 2014), the *Special Educational Needs and Disability Code of Practice, 0 to 25 Years* (Department for Education and Department of Health and Social Care, 2015), *Working Together to Safeguard Children* (Department for Education, 2026), statutory relationships and health education guidance, and (for online harms) the Online Safety Act 2023 (Great Britain, 2023) and the Office of Communications' child safety framework (Office of Communications, 2025).

This safeguarding dimension is reinforced by *Keeping Children Safe in Education 2025* (Department for Education, 2025a), which provides statutory guidance for schools and colleges on safeguarding children and safer recruitment. Read alongside *Preventing and Tackling Bullying* (Department for Education, 2017), it makes clear that bullying, including cyberbullying and prejudice-based harm, should be understood within wider safeguarding and child protection responsibilities, rather than treated only as a behavioural issue.

Taken together, these frameworks show that bullying is not treated in policy as a standalone behavioural issue, but as a matter of conduct, safety, equality, inclusion, the curriculum and child protection.

The first responsibility of policymakers is therefore to establish bullying as a public health, educational and safeguarding priority rather than a minor disciplinary concern. National or regional anti-bullying frameworks should bring together education departments, health services, social care, youth services, online safety bodies and inspectorates. This kind of joined-up approach matters because bullying does not only affect school behaviour. It affects attendance, mental health, help-seeking, belonging and, in some cases, long-term educational engagement. Fragmented systems tend to produce fragmented responses, where schools are expected to manage complex harm with limited access to external support. A stronger policy response would integrate prevention, early identification, targeted support and recovery pathways across agencies rather than locating responsibility in one sector alone (WHO Regional Office for Europe, 2024).

Second, policymakers should require schools to have clear anti-bullying measures, but should avoid assuming that the existence of a policy document is evidence of effective practice.

In England, *Preventing and Tackling Bullying* (Department for Education, 2017) states that every school must have measures in place to prevent all forms of bullying, and that, for maintained schools, these measures must form part of the behaviour policy communicated to pupils, school staff and parents under section 89 of the Education and Inspections Act 2006 (Great Britain, 2006). *Behaviour in Schools* (Department for Education, 2024) reinforces that expectation by situating anti-bullying practice within the school's wider behaviour framework and by applying that guidance across the full range of school types.

However, policy presence is not the same as policy quality. Kidwai and Smith's content analysis of 200 anti-bullying policies in England found that, on average, school policies contained only 61 percent of the items in their scoring framework. Fewer than a quarter referred to the responsibilities of non-teaching staff, guidance for parents, support for children who bully to change their behaviour, or specific powers relating to cyberbullying and out-of-school bullying. Although better policy coverage was associated with lower self-reported victimisation and perpetration, these relationships were negative, but very small (Kidwai and Smith, 2024). This is an important finding for policymakers because it shows that requiring schools to have a policy is necessary, but insufficient. Stronger expectations are needed around content, accessibility, implementation, review and impact.

Third, policymakers should fund implementation, not simply policy statements. A recurring weakness in anti-bullying policy is that governments endorse broad principles, but fail to provide the infrastructure needed to turn them into routine practice. Lekamge et al. (2025), in a systematic review and meta-analysis of whole-school interventions, found significant reductions in cyberbullying, cyber aggression and regular smoking, but also concluded that many non-significant findings were likely related to a suboptimal translation of the Health Promoting Schools Framework into practice, and inadequate sensitivity to local developmental needs. Their review is particularly useful because it shows that effective whole-school work is not a single lesson or campaign, but a coordinated framework involving curriculum, the social and physical environment, leadership, policy and resourcing, partnerships, health services and government-level support (Lekamge et al., 2025). For policymakers, the implication is clear. If implementation is under-resourced, impact will remain inconsistent.

This means that national strategies should provide sustained investment in workforce development, staff training, implementation support, data systems and access to specialist services. Schools cannot be expected to deliver complex anti-bullying work without time, expertise and referral pathways.

Preventing and Tackling Bullying (Department for Education, 2017) itself recognises that schools should involve parents, monitor bullying incidents consistently, respond to bullying outside the school gates where appropriate, and consider underlying needs, including special educational needs and disabilities, and vulnerability. Yet, such expectations are unlikely to be met consistently where staffing, pastoral capacity, educational psychology input and links with mental health services are weak.

Fourth, policymakers should build accountability around meaningful outcomes rather than relying on compliance indicators alone. In practice, many systems still judge schools too narrowly, asking whether a policy exists, whether incidents are recorded, or whether a programme has been delivered. These measures are not irrelevant, but are incomplete. Policy should also require evidence that children feel safer, are more likely to seek help, trust adults to respond, and remain engaged with the school. The Department for Education's guidance is explicit that inspectors are interested in the impact of a school's actions, not simply the recording of bullying incidents (Department for Education, 2017). This is consistent with wider evidence suggesting that school climate, belonging and perceived safety are important outcomes in their own right. Positive teacher–student relationships are associated with belonging, engagement, attendance and wellbeing, while a positive school climate, including school safety and fairness of rules, is associated with lower bullying and victimisation trajectories over time (Nix et al., 2022; Marchante et al., 2022). Policymakers should therefore require monitoring frameworks that include school belonging, perceived safety, reporting confidence, attendance and subgroup disparities alongside incident data.

Fifth, anti-bullying policy must be explicitly inclusive. Universal approaches are important, but they are not enough if they fail to reach those at greater risk. The evidence reviewed elsewhere in this chapter shows that pupils with special educational needs and disabilities are disproportionately affected by bullying, yet intervention research often fails to include them adequately or examine subgroup outcomes. Policymakers should therefore require anti-bullying frameworks to align with equality duties, accessibility standards and inclusive design principles from the outset. This includes accessible reporting routes, the adaptation of materials and communication, staff training in disability and vulnerability, and targeted support where needed. This legal and policy position is already reflected in England's school framework. *Preventing and Tackling Bullying* (Department for Education, 2017) explains that maintained schools and academies are required to comply with the Public Sector Equality Duty under the Equality Act 2010 (Great Britain, 2010), and that schools also have duties under Part 3 of the Children and Families Act 2014 (Great Britain, 2014) to ensure that pupils with special educational needs engage in school activities alongside peers without special educational needs and disabilities. *Behaviour in Schools* (Department for Education, 2024) further states that staff should ensure that the Children and Families Act 2014, the Equality Act 2010, and regulations under those Acts are complied with. In practice, this means that anti-bullying systems should be designed with accessibility, reasonable adjustment, participation and equality duties in mind from the outset, not added retrospectively once a problem becomes visible.

Sixth, policymakers should recognise that cyberbullying requires action beyond the school gate. The WHO report identifies virtual peer violence as an urgent priority, and the Department for Education's guidance makes clear that schools should investigate incidents reported outside school premises or online and take appropriate action (Department for Education, 2017; WHO Regional Office for Europe, 2024). National responses therefore need to connect education policy with wider online safety regulation, safeguarding duties and digital citizenship education. Schools can teach respectful online behaviour and reporting, but governments and regulators also have responsibilities in relation to platform design, safety expectations and legal protections. Where cyberbullying is treated as a purely school-based issue, policy will remain structurally too weak for the scale of the harm.

Finally, policymakers should be realistic about the evidence base, while still acting decisively. Anti-bullying work should be evidence-informed, but it should not be reduced to the assumption that one branded programme will solve the problem in every context. Bozic and Gutzwiller-Helfenfinger (2023) argue that internationally funded and non-governmental organization (NGO)-led anti-bullying programmes often involve important collaborative and preventive activity, but may struggle with sustainability, rigorous evaluation, local ownership, and the gap between reported activity and evidence of effectiveness. Their analysis suggests that policymakers should support evidence-informed, context-sensitive, whole-education approaches rather than short-term, under-evaluated initiatives that cannot easily be sustained once project funding ends. This is particularly important in systems where local implementation capacity varies widely.

In summary, the policy task is not simply to tell schools to tackle bullying more effectively. It is to build the conditions in which effective prevention and response become possible. That means clear statutory expectations, stronger accountability, sustained funding, inclusive design, integration with health and safeguarding systems, and serious attention to digital harms. It also means accepting that good policy is not measured by how comprehensive it appears on paper, but by whether children feel safer, more supported and more confident that, when harm occurs, adults will act.

What Education Systems and Schools Should Do

Schools remain central to any serious anti-bullying strategy, but the evidence suggests they are most effective when bullying prevention is embedded within the wider culture of the school rather than treated as an isolated behavioural issue. This matters because bullying does not emerge only from individual pupil behaviour. It is shaped by peer norms, clarity of expectations, the consistency of adult response, the quality of teacher–pupil relationships, the ease of reporting and whether children feel that they belong in school. Where anti-bullying work is reduced to a policy document, an annual assembly or a reactive disciplinary process, schools may be able to demonstrate activity without necessarily improving pupils' daily experience of safety and inclusion. By contrast, schools that succeed tend to create environments in which respect, fairness and support are visible in everyday practice, across classrooms, corridors, playgrounds, transport routes and online interactions. This whole-school emphasis is consistent with the Health Promoting Schools Framework, which conceptualises effective prevention as change across curriculum, ethos and environment, school governance, policy and resourcing, school and community partnerships, school health services and wider governmental support (Lekamge et al., 2025).

One of the clearest implications for schools is that anti-bullying work should be integrated into the broader behaviour, safeguarding and inclusion framework of the institution. In England, *Behaviour in Schools* (Department for Education, 2024) makes clear that schools should develop a behaviour policy that promotes good behaviour and applies across maintained schools, academies, free schools, non-maintained special schools and independent schools, while *Keeping Children Safe in Education* (Department for Education, 2025a) sets out the legal duties schools and colleges must follow to safeguard and promote the welfare of children. Taken together, these frameworks make clear that bullying should not be treated as a standalone pastoral issue. It sits within behaviour, child protection, attendance, inclusion and wider school safety. Anti-bullying practice, therefore, should be embedded in the school's wider approach to conduct, reporting, support and safeguarding rather than operating as an isolated initiative.

However, even the best written policy cannot compensate for a weak school climate. Research increasingly suggests that belonging, fairness, safety and relational trust are not secondary outcomes, but part of the mechanism through which bullying is prevented and recovery becomes possible. Nix et al.'s systematic quantitative review found that positive teacher–student relationships support students' work habits, engagement, wellbeing, attendance and sense of belonging at school, and identified fairness, engagement and achievement as key themes in the literature (Nix et al., 2022). This has direct relevance for anti-bullying work. If children experience school as a place where they are respected, included and supported, the social conditions that sustain bullying are weakened. The converse is also true. Where relationships are poor, rules feel arbitrary and some pupils feel persistently marginal or unseen, bullying may flourish beneath the surface even when formal policies exist. Schools should therefore treat belonging and relational safety as core prevention targets. This means paying attention not only to what is taught, but to how teachers interact with pupils, how conflict is managed, how inclusion is enacted, and whether pupils experience adults as fair, available and trustworthy.

The role of school safety and climate is further reinforced by Williams et al. (2018), who found that, in a public high school sample, 24.7 percent of students reported feeling unsafe and 14.4 percent reported avoiding school because they felt unsafe. After accounting for bullying victimisation, students felt safer when they reported positive student and teacher relationships, more consistent rules, a better physical environment and a stronger sense of school belonging. School avoidance due to feeling unsafe was more strongly associated with lower belonging and poorer teacher relationships than with bullying itself in the final model (Williams et al., 2018). This is a powerful finding for education professionals because it shows that reducing bullying incidents is not the only relevant aim. Schools should also ask whether children feel safe enough to attend, participate and remain connected to learning. Measures of belonging, perceived safety and attendance, therefore, have a legitimate place within anti-bullying evaluation and school improvement.

Schools should also recognise that some periods and spaces require additional attention. Transition points are particularly important. Marchante et al. (2022) found that, during the transition into middle school, more positive trajectories in teacher–student relationships, student–student relationships, school safety and liking of school were associated with more positive victimisation trajectories, while fairness of rules was associated with bullying trajectories. Their study highlights how changes in school climate during transition can shape pupils' risk of victimisation and points to the value of transition support, mentoring and whole-school transition programmes involving teachers, staff, parents and older pupils (Marchante et al., 2022). For schools, this suggests that anti-bullying work should not be distributed evenly across the year without regard to context. Entry into a new school, movement between key stages, and other periods of social instability may require intensified relational support, orientation work, peer mentoring and visible staff presence. It also suggests that schools should pay close attention to fairness of rules and school safety, both of which are likely to affect how pupils interpret the legitimacy and trustworthiness of the environment they are entering.

A further implication is that schools must make disclosure easier, not simply encourage it in principle. Help-seeking cannot be assumed. Grüne and Willems (2024) found that, among bullied adolescents, 60 percent sought help, but only 32 percent of those sought formal help, while most sought help from family and friends. Family cohesion and self-efficacy were positively associated with help-seeking. This indicates that schools cannot assume pupils will naturally disclose to staff or use formal reporting systems. If children doubt that adults will take them seriously, fear retaliation or feel ashamed, significant harm may remain hidden. Reporting mechanisms therefore need to be clear, visible and emotionally safe. Schools should provide more than one route to disclosure, including trusted adults, anonymous systems where appropriate, pastoral routes and digital reporting where needed. They should also make explicit what happens after a report is made, because uncertainty can deter help-seeking as much as fear. Pupils need to know that they will be listened to, that action will follow, and that reporting will not worsen their situation.

The quality of adult response is equally important. Gizzarelli et al. (2023) found that staff responses to student reports of bullying could include no response at all, and that staff preparedness predicted staff involvement following bullying incidents. Their review also found that strategies to improve responses included whole-school anti-bullying programmes and training to increase staff efficacy. This is highly relevant to schools because it shows that a reporting system is only as effective as the adults who receive the report. Staff need training not only in recognising bullying, but in responding promptly, proportionately and consistently. They need confidence in handling covert, as well as overt bullying, clarity about referral routes and support from leadership. They also need to understand that dismissive or inconsistent responses can have system-wide consequences, because one poor response may reduce future reporting from the child involved and from their peers. In this respect, staff development should be seen as a safeguarding and inclusion issue, not merely a behavioural training exercise.

Schools should also work more deliberately with families. *Preventing and Tackling Bullying* (Department for Education, 2017) makes it clear that successful schools involve parents, ensure that they understand school procedures, and build confidence that concerns will be taken seriously. This is supported by evidence from Lester et al. (2017), whose study of the Friendly Schools Friendly Families intervention found that parents exposed to the parent component reported significant increases in discussions with their child about bullying, and that a parent intervention can improve parent–child communication when embedded within a whole-school approach. Similarly, Chen et al. (2021) conclude that parenting components can contribute to bullying reduction, strengthen parent–child communication and enhance parenting skills, while also pointing to the importance of school–family partnerships. Taken together, these findings suggest that parental involvement should not be limited to notification after an incident. Schools should provide guidance, invite meaningful communication, link home activities with classroom work where appropriate, and involve parents in prevention, as well as response.

Finally, education systems and individual schools must ensure that anti-bullying practice is inclusive. *Preventing and Tackling Bullying* (Department for Education, 2017) makes clear that schools must take account of vulnerable pupils and those with special educational needs and disabilities, while England's wider legal framework, including the Equality Act 2010, the Children and Families Act 2014 and the *Special Educational Needs and Disbility Code of Practice*, reinforces the expectation that support should be fair, accessible and responsive to additional need. In practice, this means more than acknowledging vulnerability in principle. Schools should consider whether reporting routes are accessible, whether materials and assemblies are understandable for pupils with communication differences, whether bullying linked to disability, race, religion, sexuality or other protected characteristics is explicitly addressed, and whether reasonable adjustments are built into support plans. They should also avoid responses that effectively remove the pupil who has been bullied from the school community without tackling the conditions that made school feel unsafe in the first place. *Preventing and Tackling Bullying* (Department for Education, 2017) is clear that removing bullied children from school, even temporarily, can disrupt education and send the wrong message, and that support should go hand in hand with measures to tackle the bullying so that pupils feel safe at school, and on the way to and from school.

The guidance of the Department for Education is clear that removing bullied children from school, even temporarily, can disrupt education and send the wrong message, and that support should go hand in hand with measures to tackle the bullying so that pupils feel safe at school, and on the way to and from school (Department for Education, 2017). The educational response must therefore be both protective and restorative, maintaining access to learning, while actively rebuilding safety, trust and belonging.

Overall, the educational task is not simply to respond once bullying has occurred. It is to organise the school in ways that make bullying less likely to flourish, easier to disclose and more consistently addressed when it does occur. That requires clear policies, strong relationships, fair rules, parent partnerships, trained staff and a school climate in which safety and belonging are experienced rather than merely stated. Where schools can achieve this, anti-bullying work becomes part of the everyday architecture of a safe and inclusive learning environment rather than a separate initiative layered on top of it.

Inclusion, Special Educational Needs and Disability-responsive Practice

Any serious anti-bullying strategy must recognise that bullying is not experienced equally across the pupil population. Children and young people with special educational needs and disabilities, and children with disabilities more broadly, face a disproportionate burden of victimisation and often encounter additional barriers in recognising, reporting and escaping bullying. For this reason, inclusion cannot be treated as a minor add-on to mainstream anti-bullying work. It must be built into the design, delivery and evaluation of prevention and response from the outset. Badger et al. (2024) note that pupils with special educational needs and disabilities experience bullying involvement at markedly higher rates than their peers, with self-reported victimisation in some studies estimated at two to four times higher than for pupils without special educational needs and disabilities. Their review also highlights that special educational needs and disabilities status itself, along with associated communication, social or behavioural differences, can increase vulnerability to targeting.

This matters because generic anti-bullying approaches cannot simply be assumed to work equally well for all pupils. Eldred et al. (2025) make this point clearly in their review of school-based violence prevention interventions for children with disabilities. They found that, although randomised controlled trials of school violence prevention exist, the majority did not mention children with disabilities at all. Of the few that did, only a very small number undertook subgroup analysis or described adaptations to intervention or research design. The authors therefore argue that school-based violence prevention efforts are unlikely to be genuinely successful at scale if children with disabilities are not adequately considered in either programme content or evaluation design (Eldred et al., 2025). This is an important challenge to universalist assumptions. It suggests that anti-bullying work that appears effective in the general population may still fail some of the children most at risk.

For schools and education systems, the first implication is that inclusive anti-bullying work should begin with the recognition of difference rather than expecting pupils with special educational needs and disabilities to fit into pre-existing models of delivery. Badger et al. (2024) found that there remain only a limited number of anti-bullying programmes designed or adapted specifically for pupils with special educational needs and disabilities, and although some studies reported reductions in bullying involvement, the overall evidence base was variable and often methodologically weak. Importantly, they recommend that anti-bullying programmes for pupils with special educational needs and disabilities should be co-developed with pupils, parents and staff, and should incorporate design features that support effective delivery, engagement and learning. This is especially valuable because it shifts the emphasis from simply identifying vulnerability to designing more usable and meaningful interventions.

Co-development is particularly important because bullying may look different, be interpreted differently, and be reported differently for pupils with special educational needs and disabilities. Badger et al. (2024) argue that current measures often treat bullying as a generic construct, yet reporting and experience may differ for pupils with special educational needs and disabilities or within special school settings. Some pupils may find it harder to recognise subtle relational aggression, to communicate what has happened, or to use standard reporting systems confidently. Others may be more likely to be misunderstood by adults, particularly if distress is interpreted through the lens of behaviour rather than victimisation. This means that schools should consider whether their reporting routes, investigation processes and support plans are genuinely accessible. It also means researchers and policymakers should be cautious about assuming that low disclosure reflects low prevalence. In some cases, it may instead reflect barriers to communication, social understanding or trust.

A genuinely inclusive approach therefore requires adaptation at multiple levels. Eldred et al. (2025) recommend accessible content and communication, including simplified language, visual support, augmentative and alternative communication, and more inclusive promotional materials. They also recommend adapting school environments and training delivery staff so that violence prevention work is meaningful for children with different impairments. In addition, they suggest that programmes should address drivers of violence that may be especially relevant to children with disabilities, such as stigma, social isolation and disability-targeted abuse. These recommendations are highly relevant to bullying prevention because they move inclusion beyond the narrow idea of physical access and towards a fuller model of cognitive, communicative and social accessibility.

The review by Eldred et al. (2025) is also valuable because it proposes a twin-track approach. This means adapting mainstream interventions so that children with disabilities can benefit from universal provision, while also developing targeted interventions for disability-specific or disability-targeted forms of violence where necessary. This is a particularly helpful framework for schools and policymakers because it avoids a false choice between inclusion and specialist support. Mainstream anti-bullying work should be accessible to all, but it may still need to be supplemented by bespoke approaches for some pupils, particularly where communication needs, sensory needs or specific patterns of abuse require a more tailored response. For example, children with intellectual or communication disabilities may need additional reporting mechanisms, greater adult mediation or more structured support to understand peer intent and social safety.

Schools should also pay attention to where and how pupils with special educational needs and disabilities are educated. Badger et al. (2024) note evidence suggesting that pupils with special educational needs and disabilities in inclusive education settings may be less involved in bullying than those in more segregated settings, although comparison data remain limited and interpretation is complex. This does not mean that inclusion alone protects against bullying, but it does suggest that separation can, in some cases, intensify visibility, difference or social vulnerability. The implication is not that one setting is universally safer than another, but that schools should be alert to how structures, peer culture and adult expectations shape risk. Inclusive education must therefore be accompanied by deliberate relational work, anti-stigma education, staff training and peer culture interventions if it is to offer genuine protection.

An inclusive anti-bullying response must also avoid approaches that inadvertently punish or marginalise the child who is being harmed. Pupils with special educational needs and disabilities may already experience exclusion, misunderstanding or increased adult surveillance. If the school response to bullying results in the pupil being removed from shared spaces, over-restricted or quietly separated without wider change, then the burden of adjustment falls once again on the child who has been targeted. Instead, support plans should aim to rebuild safety, while maintaining access to learning, relationships and participation. That may include adapted check-ins, trusted adults, supported peer networks, visual reporting tools, predictable routines and reasonable adjustments during investigation and recovery. The goal should not be mere containment, but meaningful reintegration into a school environment that feels safer and more trustworthy.

Overall, the evidence suggests that anti-bullying work for pupils with special educational needs and disabilities should not be treated as a specialist concern at the margins of school policy. It should be understood as a test of whether anti-bullying systems are genuinely equitable. If prevention programmes, reporting routes and support structures are designed only with the most communicatively confident and socially typical pupils in mind, they will fail precisely those children who may need protection most. Inclusion, therefore, requires more than acknowledgement. It requires co-design, accessibility, adaptation, targeted support where needed and a more rigorous evaluation of whether existing approaches are truly working for all pupils.

What Health and Mental Health Professionals Should Do

Health and mental health professionals play an important role in anti-bullying work, yet they are often positioned at the margins of prevention policy, with schools remaining the default site of responsibility. This is too narrow. Bullying and cyberbullying are increasingly recognised as public health issues because they contribute to psychological distress, social difficulties, developmental harm and reduced wellbeing across childhood and adolescence. Dailey et al. (2025) argue that healthcare and public health professionals are uniquely placed to contribute to early identification, prevention, resilience-building and recovery, but that their roles are not consistently integrated into anti-bullying frameworks. Their review is especially useful because it shows that health-led responses are not limited to treatment after harm has occurred. They can also strengthen prevention, family support, cross-sector collaboration and more timely recognition of distress.

One of the clearest implications for practice is that bullying should be considered routinely when children and young people present with anxiety, low mood, school avoidance, somatic complaints, social withdrawal, self-harm or distress linked to peer relationships. Dailey et al. (2025) identify screening and early identification as one of the six core themes in healthcare and public health interventions. They note that clinicians, school nurses and allied health professionals often encounter bullying-related distress in practice, yet standardised definitions, screening tools and referral protocols remain underdeveloped. This is important because young people do not always disclose bullying spontaneously, and formal help-seeking remains limited. Health professionals therefore need to ask about peer relationships and bullying directly, rather than waiting for the child or family to volunteer this information. In practical terms, this means incorporating bullying-related questions into psychosocial assessments, school health reviews, safeguarding conversations and mental health triage where appropriate.

A further implication is that support should be multidisciplinary and trauma-informed. Dailey et al. (2025) identify family and community involvement, multi-component school-based interventions, cognitive behavioural and solution-focused approaches, and online or digital interventions as key themes within the health-led literature. They conclude that the strongest approaches are those that extend beyond the individual and connect children with supportive adults across home, school and community contexts. This is highly relevant for bullying because the harm is relational and often sustained across settings. Children who are being bullied may need more than individual coping advice. They may require help to rebuild a sense of safety, restore confidence in adults, improve emotional regulation, strengthen peer support and re-establish school engagement. Trauma-informed care is especially important where bullying has been chronic, humiliating or accompanied by significant anxiety, avoidance or dysregulation. In these cases, professionals should respond in ways that emphasise safety, collaboration, empowerment and predictable support rather than inadvertently reproducing blame, disbelief or fragmentation.

Health professionals should also work more deliberately with families. Family and community engagement emerges repeatedly in the literature as a protective and implementation-enhancing factor. Dailey et al. (2025)

found that interventions involving caregivers were generally associated with stronger engagement, more consistent follow-through and greater potential for longer-term behavioural change at home and in school. Their review describes structured outreach, caregiver psychoeducation, family communication work and community partnerships as recurring features of more effective programmes. For practitioners, this means that assessment and intervention should not stop with the child alone. Parents and carers may need help to understand the impact of bullying, respond supportively, communicate with schools and reinforce coping strategies or recovery plans at home. This is particularly important where children are reluctant to disclose formally at school, because families may be the first or only source of help sought. Health professionals are therefore well placed to bridge the gap between the child's emotional experience, family understanding and school response.

There is also a growing case for using digital and hybrid forms of support, particularly where bullying involves online spaces or where access to face-to-face services is limited. Dailey et al. (2025) describe digital and hybrid interventions as promising, but under-used, with potential to expand access to coping strategies, psychoeducation and support beyond the traditional school setting. They note that such approaches may be especially relevant for dispersed or underserved populations and for young people who are more comfortable engaging through digital modes. This does not mean that digital interventions should replace relational care, but it does suggest that health systems and school-linked services should consider how online tools, structured self-help, digital screening or hybrid support models might complement more traditional approaches. Given the role of cyberbullying in contemporary peer harm, the ability of health professionals to work confidently across both in-person and online contexts is likely to become increasingly important.

At the same time, the evidence base for recovery-focused interventions remains more limited than the evidence for identification and multi-component prevention. Al-Alawi et al. (2025) - found that psychoeducational interventions showed a small, but significant effect in reducing social isolation and loneliness among school pupils, but there were not enough publications to conduct a meta-analysis of effects on post-traumatic stress symptoms. Their review concludes that psychoeducational approaches show promise, but that further research is needed to determine optimal implementation, and understand their effects more fully. This is an important caution. It suggests that professionals should avoid overstating what is known, particularly in relation to trauma-related outcomes, while still recognising that structured psychosocial support may help address some of the relational and emotional consequences of bullying. In practice, this means that interventions should be individualised, monitored and linked to ongoing assessment rather than delivered as though any one model will work for all young people.

Finally, health and mental health professionals also play an advocacy role. Dailey et al. (2025) emphasise that implementation remains constrained by insufficient training, workload pressures, limited institutional support, fragmented coordination between health and education systems, and lack of protected time for delivery. These barriers are not minor operational issues. They shape whether children receive timely, joined-up support or fall between services. Professionals working in paediatrics, school nursing, primary care, Child and Adolescent Mental Health Services (CAMHS), counselling, educational psychology and public health can therefore contribute not only through direct clinical work, but by advocating for structured referral pathways, protected training time, trauma-informed practice, and stronger integration between schools and health systems. In this sense, the task is not merely to respond once distress has become severe. It is to help build a service landscape in which bullying-related harm is recognised earlier, addressed more coherently, and less likely to become a hidden driver of longer-term mental health difficulty.

Cyberbullying and Digital Harm

Cyberbullying now requires explicit attention within any serious anti-bullying strategy because it changes the scale, reach and persistence of harm. Unlike many in-person incidents, digital abuse can occur at any time of day, may be repeated rapidly, and can be shared with a potentially much wider audience. The WHO Health Behaviour in School-aged Children report identifies cyberbullying as an urgent priority, noting that virtual forms of peer violence became increasingly relevant as young people's social worlds shifted online and that cyberbullying must now be viewed as a major issue for societies, not simply for individual schools (WHO Regional Office for Europe, 2024). The same report found that one in eight adolescents reported cyberbullying, others at least once or twice in the previous couple of months, and that 15 percent reported being cyberbullied, with the increase in victimisation particularly concerning among younger girls (WHO Regional Office for Europe, 2024). These patterns underline the fact that digital harm is not peripheral to contemporary bullying prevention, but central to it.

Cyberbullying also requires a policy response that goes beyond schools alone. The Online Safety Act 2023 (Great Britain, 2023) received Royal Assent on 26 October 2023 and now places legal duties on social media companies and search services to protect children and adults online. GOV.UK guidance states that, from 25 July 2025, platforms must protect children from harmful and age-inappropriate content, including bullying, and must provide clear and accessible ways for children and parents to report problems when they arise. The Office of Communications, as the independent regulator, has enforcement powers to assess and enforce compliance. This matters because some of the drivers of cyberbullying, including rapid sharing, amplification and platform design, lie beyond the control of schools and families alone.

Cyberbullying also deserves distinct treatment because its mechanisms differ in important ways from traditional bullying. *Preventing and Tackling Bullying* (Department for Education, 2017) describes cyberbullying as a form of virtual bullying that can occur both in and outside school, at all times of the day, with a potentially larger audience and greater opportunities for harmful material to be forwarded and recirculated quickly (Department for Education, 2017). Dailey et al., (2025) similarly argue that cyberbullying adds complexity because anonymity, persistence and wide reach can intensify psychological harm and reduce the victim's sense of escape or safety. This means that children may remain exposed long after the original act, including in spaces that should ordinarily offer respite, such as the home. It also means that humiliation, exclusion, threats and reputational harm may become more enduring and more difficult for adults to detect. In practice, digital aggression often overlaps with in-person peer dynamics rather than replacing them, but its amplification effects make it especially damaging.

For policymakers and schools, one implication is that cyberbullying cannot be treated as something outside educational responsibility simply because it occurs online or beyond school hours. *Preventing and Tackling Bullying* (Department for Education, 2017) is explicit that if an incident of bullying outside the school premises or online is reported to the school, it should be investigated and appropriate action taken. The guidance also notes that schools should make it easy for pupils to report bullying that may have occurred outside the school, including cyberbullying, and should update their approach in light of technological developments (Department for Education, 2017). This is important because digital harm does not stop mattering once it crosses the school gate. If schools respond only to incidents that occur physically on site, they risk ignoring some of the most pervasive and psychologically intrusive forms of peer abuse now experienced by children and young people.

At the same time, schools should not be expected to carry the full burden alone. Cyberbullying sits at the intersection of education, parenting, safeguarding, health and online platform governance. The WHO report calls for the education of young people, families and schools about the forms and implications of cyberbullying, while also recognising the need to regulate social media platforms in order to limit exposure (WHO Regional Office for Europe, 2024). This wider framing matters because some of the drivers of cyberbullying, including rapid sharing, anonymity, algorithmic amplification and platform design, lie beyond the control of schools and individual families. A credible response therefore requires coordination across sectors, including digital literacy education, family guidance, school reporting systems, safeguarding pathways and stronger expectations of online environments.

Recent health and public health literature points in the same direction. Dailey et al. (2025) identify online and digital interventions as one of the six core themes in their systematic review of bullying and cyberbullying interventions involving healthcare and public health professionals. They note that digital approaches, including web-based modules, online cognitive behavioural interventions and virtual counselling, may improve access, reduce barriers and extend support beyond the traditional school setting. They also identify digital citizenship training, interactive skill-building and caregiver-focused content as recurring features of promising interventions. Importantly, however, they also point to a consistent implementation gap, with health-led digital interventions often operating in isolation rather than being integrated into broader health or public health systems (Dailey et al., 2025). For practice, this means that digital tools may be valuable, but they work best when they complement, rather than replace, coordinated relational support from schools, families and services.

Schools also need to ensure that their policies explicitly cover cyberbullying and related powers. Kidwai and Smith (2024) found that, although policy coverage in England had improved over time, only a minority of school anti-bullying policies discussed specific powers and strategies to deal with cyberbullying and out-of-school bullying. They argue that policies should be more explicit about the powers available to schools, and clearer in their practical guidance to parents and the wider school community. This is a particularly useful point because it shows that cyberbullying is now widely recognised in principle, yet is often still underdeveloped in operational policy. A school may claim to address cyberbullying without making clear how staff should respond, what happens when incidents take place outside school hours, what parents should do, or how evidence from devices and online platforms should be handled. A stronger digital harms policy therefore requires not only recognition, but practical clarity.

In educational terms, the most effective response to cyberbullying is likely to be preventive, relational and developmental. This includes teaching digital citizenship, empathy, consent, respectful communication and the risks of rapid sharing, making reporting easy and credible, involving parents in understanding online harm, and ensuring that staff are trained to respond proportionately and confidently. This is consistent with the statutory *Relationships Education, Relationships and Sex Education (RSE) and Health Education* (Department for Education, 2025b) guidance, which was updated in December 2025 for introduction from 1 September 2026 and applies across schools in England. The guidance provides the curriculum basis for teaching respectful relationships, safety and help-seeking as part of wider health and relationships education. Dailey et al. (2025) reinforce this by highlighting empathy training, caregiver education, coping strategies and collaboration between schools, families and health professionals as important components in reducing cyberbullying and promoting wellbeing. Taken together, these findings suggest that cyberbullying prevention should not sit in a narrow online safety box. It should form part of a broader educational approach to relationships, responsibility, resilience and help-seeking in a digital age.

Implementation, Evaluation and Accountability

One of the clearest themes running through the contemporary literature is that anti-bullying work often falters not because schools or policymakers lack intentions, but because implementation is inconsistent, under-supported or assessed too narrowly. In practice, there remains a tendency to treat anti-bullying action as complete once a policy has been published, a programme has been purchased, or a staff training day has taken place. The evidence suggests that this is not enough. Kidwai and Smith (2024) found that, although policy coverage in England had improved over time, school policies still varied substantially in scope and quality, with an average coverage of 61 percent across their scoring framework. They also found that correlations between overall policy score and self-reported victimisation and perpetration were negative, but very small, indicating that policy quality alone has, at best, only a limited relationship with behavioural outcomes. This is an important finding for this chapter because it demonstrates that written policy is necessary, but cannot be treated as a proxy for real-world protection or culture change.

This problem is not confined to policy documents. It extends to programme delivery and wider systems design. The wider intervention literature increasingly shows that anti-bullying work is highly sensitive to how well approaches are implemented, adapted and sustained. As other sections of this chapter have shown, whole-school interventions appear most promising when they are embedded within broader changes to school climate, relationships, leadership and support systems rather than delivered as isolated activities. The practical implication is that implementation should be treated as a central part of anti-bullying strategy rather than as an administrative afterthought. Schools need time, leadership support, workforce capacity and opportunities for reflection if prevention work is to become part of daily practice rather than a short-lived initiative.

A useful way of understanding this is to distinguish between delivery and implementation. Delivery asks whether an activity took place. Implementation asks whether it was understood, accepted, accessible, sustained and integrated into the school's routine life. A school may be able to show that it delivered an assembly, revised a policy, or introduced an online reporting form, yet still failed to change pupils' day-to-day experience of safety or support. For this reason, implementation should include attention to acceptability, fidelity, adaptation and reach. This is especially important where schools serve diverse pupil populations, including pupils with special educational needs and disabilities, because an approach that is delivered in a generic form may not be experienced as usable or protective by those most at risk. Badger et al. (2024) note that few studies evaluating anti-bullying approaches for pupils with special educational needs and disabilities report adequately on feasibility or social validity, meaning that it often remains unclear whether interventions are genuinely acceptable and workable for staff, pupils and parents.

Evaluation should therefore move beyond the question of whether a school has done something and ask whether what was done was meaningful. This requires a broader and more sophisticated set of indicators. Incident counts remain useful, but they cannot be the only measure of success. Policies and programmes may increase reporting in the short term, particularly where pupils become more confident that adults will take them seriously. In such cases, a rise in recorded incidents may reflect improved trust rather than worsening behaviour. Conversely, low reporting may reflect fear, poor systems or weak adult credibility rather than genuine safety. Grüne and Willems (2024) show why this matters. Among bullied adolescents in their study, 60 percent sought help, but only 32 percent of those sought formal help, with most turning instead to family and friends. This suggests that formal reporting systems are often used by a minority, even when harm is present, and that schools cannot assume that silence means the absence of bullying.

For this reason, accountability frameworks should include not only prevalence and incident data, but also measures of reporting confidence, adult responsiveness, belonging, school safety and attendance. Nix et al. (2022) demonstrate that positive teacher–student relationships are associated with wellbeing, attendance, inclusion and belonging, while Williams et al. (2018) show that perceptions of school safety and school avoidance are shaped by teacher relationships, rule consistency, the physical environment and a sense of belonging, not simply by bullying victimisation alone. Together, these findings support the view that anti-bullying work should be judged partly by whether pupils feel safe enough to attend, participate in and seek help. A school that records fewer bullying incidents, but still has pupils who feel unsafe, avoid school or distrust adults cannot reasonably be described as successful.

The quality of adult response is another critical accountability issue. If schools encourage disclosure, but respond inconsistently, pupils may quickly learn that formal reporting offers little protection. Gizzarelli et al. (2023) found that school staff responses to student reports of bullying could include no response at all, and that staff preparedness was a predictor of staff involvement following bullying incidents. Their review also found that strategies to improve responses included whole-school anti-bullying programmes and training to increase staff efficacy. At the same time, they stress that the evidence base itself is limited, with relatively few studies examining real-life responses to actual student reports rather than hypothetical scenarios. This is a valuable reminder that implementation should be evaluated not only from the perspective of institutional procedure, but also from the perspective of pupils. Do children believe staff will act? Are responses timely and proportionate? Do adults follow up? Are pupils left feeling safer afterwards? These are practical accountability questions, not optional additions.

There is also a strong case for evaluating how implementation functions at key transition points and within changing school climates. Marchante et al.

(2022) found that more positive trajectories in teacher–student relationships, student–student relationships, school safety and liking of school during the transition to middle school were associated with more positive victimisation trajectories. They argue that intervention programmes should involve the whole-school community and address social, academic and logistical factors during transition. This is highly relevant to implementation because it shows that timing and context matter. Anti-bullying work may need to be intensified or adapted during school transition, when friendship structures are shifting, younger pupils are more vulnerable, and perceptions of fairness and safety may change quickly. Accountability should therefore consider whether support is responsive to developmental periods rather than delivered in a flat and uniform manner throughout the school year.

Another issue is who owns the work. Bozic and Gutzwiller-Helfenfinger (2023) argue that anti-bullying programmes, especially where supported by external agencies or international actors, may be weakened by limited local ownership, insufficient monitoring or weak institutional capacity. Although their discussion is broader than school-level implementation alone, it is highly relevant here. Programmes are less likely to be sustained where they are seen as externally imposed, poorly aligned with local need, or disconnected from the realities of staff workload and school infrastructure. This suggests that accountability should include questions of ownership, leadership commitment, staff involvement and partnerships with families and pupils. Implementation is stronger when those expected to deliver or use the approach have had a role in shaping it.

The role of staff development is especially important. Training is often recommended, but not all training is equal. Gizzarelli et al. (2023) note that some studies found strong associations between whole-school programmes, staff training and greater intervention in bullying incidents, while others found weaker or mixed effects. They also report recommendations that include improving staff confidence and self-efficacy, helping teachers understand social dynamics, involving staff in policymaking, and encouraging shared responsibility across the school. This implies that professional development should not be limited to definitional awareness. It should include practical response strategies, relational work, handling covert bullying, understanding digital harm, and knowing when and how to escalate concerns. It should also be reinforced over time rather than delivered once and assumed to endure.

For policymakers, school leaders and inspectorates, the central implication is that anti-bullying accountability should be framed as a question of protective capacity. This includes whether the school has a clear and accessible policy, whether staff feel prepared, whether pupils trust adults, whether reporting routes are workable, whether vulnerable groups can access support, whether responses are followed up, and whether the wider school climate promotes safety and belonging. It also includes whether schools use their data intelligently. Recording incidents is only useful if schools analyse patterns, identify hotspots and vulnerable groups, monitor repeat incidents, and use the data to review whether their approach is working. Kidwai and Smith (2024) note that coverage of how data would be used had improved, but unevenly, reinforcing the need for better policy translation into practice.

Ultimately, implementation, evaluation and accountability should not be understood as technical exercises detached from children's lived experience. They are the means by which schools and systems determine whether their anti-bullying work is genuinely protective or merely procedural. A robust approach will therefore ask not only whether an intervention was delivered, but whether it was trusted, accessible, inclusive, well supported and capable of changing the daily conditions in which bullying occurs. Without that level of scrutiny, anti-bullying policy risks remain strongest on paper and weakest where they matter most, in the actual experience of children and young people.

Conclusion

The evidence reviewed across this chapter shows that bullying is not a minor behavioural issue that can be solved through isolated sanctions, awareness weeks or policy statements alone. It is a public health, educational, safeguarding and equity concern that requires coordinated, sustained and evidence-informed action. Recent international data show that bullying and cyberbullying remain significant concerns across adolescence, while school-based and public health research demonstrates that effective responses depend on much more than the presence of a written policy. They depend on implementation quality, staff preparedness, school climate, family engagement, inclusion and the availability of trusted routes to help (WHO Regional Office for Europe, 2024; Dailey et al., 2025; Lekamge et al., 2025).

For policymakers, the challenge is to build systems that make effective prevention and response possible. This means creating joined-up frameworks across education, health, safeguarding and digital policy, funding implementation rather than aspiration, and holding schools to account for outcomes that matter, including safety, belonging, help-seeking and equitable access to support. For education systems and schools, the task is to move anti-bullying work out of the margins of school life and into the everyday culture of the institution. Policies must be usable, staff must be prepared, pupils must trust that reports will lead to action, and families must be treated as partners rather than passive recipients of information.

The chapter also shows that inclusion must be central rather than incidental. Children with special educational needs and disabilities continue to face disproportionate risks, yet intervention design and evaluation too often fail to reflect their experiences or needs (Badger et al., 2024; Eldred et al., 2025). Likewise, cyberbullying and digital harm require anti-bullying work to extend beyond the physical school environment and engage with the realities of young people's online lives. Health and mental health professionals also have a significant role to play, not only in identifying distress and supporting recovery, but in strengthening multidisciplinary responses and advocating for earlier, more coherent support.

Perhaps the most important lesson is that anti-bullying success should not be judged only by whether a school has a policy or whether incident numbers appear to fall. It should also be judged by whether children feel safe, whether they belong, whether they seek help, and whether adults respond in ways that are timely, credible and protective (Nix et al., 2022; Gizzarelli et al., 2023; Grüne and Willems, 2024). Without this wider perspective, anti-bullying work risks becoming procedural rather than genuinely protective.

Bullying prevention and response must therefore be understood as a long-term commitment to building safer, fairer and more inclusive environments for children and young people. That requires action at every level, from national strategy and school leadership to staff development, family communication and direct support for those harmed. If this chapter has shown anything, it is that meaningful progress depends not on doing more of the same, but on building systems that children can trust.

Key Takeaways

- Bullying should be treated as a public health, educational, safeguarding and equity issue rather than a minor disciplinary problem
- Written anti-bullying policies are necessary, but policy alone has limited value without implementation, review and impact
- Whole-school approaches are most effective when they are embedded in school culture, relationships, fairness and belonging
- Children with special educational needs and disabilities must be considered from the outset through inclusive design, accessible reporting and targeted support where needed
- Parent and family engagement strengthens prevention, communication and recovery, and should form part of routine anti-bullying work
- Health and mental health professionals play an important role in screening, early identification, multidisciplinary support and advocacy
- Cyberbullying requires schools, families, health services, policymakers and digital systems to respond together rather than in isolation
- Anti-bullying success should be judged not only by incident counts, but by safety, help-seeking, belonging, attendance and the credibility of the adult response

References

Al-Alawi, K.S., Eltayib, R.A.A., Al Saadoon, M., Alhaj, A.H., Aldhafri, S., Al-Adawi, S. and Chan, M.F. (2025) 'Efficacy of psycho-educational interventions on school bullying in social isolation, loneliness and PTSD among schoolchildren: A systematic review and meta-analysis', *Child: Care, Health and Development*, 51(2), e70062. Available at: https://doi.org/10.1111/cch.70062.

Badger, J.R., Nisar, A. and Hastings, R.P. (2024) 'School-based anti-bullying approaches for children and young people with special educational needs and disabilities: A systematic review and synthesis', *Journal of Research in Special Educational Needs*, 24(3), pp. 742–757. Available at: https://doi.org/10.1111/1471-3802.12665.

Bozic, A. and Gutzwiller-Helfenfinger, E. (2023) 'International organisations, NGOs, and evidence-based programmes in preventing school violence and bullying', *Bildung und Erziehung*, 76, 246–264. Available at: www.researchgate.net/publication/373111416_International_Organisations_NGOs_and_Evidence-Based_Programmes_in_Preventing_School_Violence_and_Bullying/link/64db7b9278e40b48bd4c86ef/download?_tp=eyJjb250ZXh0Ijp7ImZpcnN0UGFnZSI6InB1YmxpY2F0aW9uIiwicGFnZSI6InB1YmxpY2F0aW9uIn19.

Chen, Q., Zhu, Y. and Chui, W.H. (2021) 'A Meta-analysis on effects of parenting programs on bullying prevention', *Trauma, Violence, & Abuse*, 22(5), pp. 1209–1220. doi: 10.1177/1524838020915619.

Dailey, S.F., Roche, R.R. and Sharkey, M.C. (2025) 'Addressing bullying and cyberbullying in public health: A systematic review of interventions for healthcare and public health professionals', *International Journal of Environmental Research and Public Health*, 22(11), 1682. Available at: https://doi.org/10.3390/ijerph22111682.

Department for Education (2017) *Preventing and tackling bullying*. London: Department for Education. Available at: www.gov.uk/government/publications/preventing-and-tackling-bullying (Accessed: 21 March 2026).

Department for Education (2024) *Behaviour in schools: Advice for headteachers and school staff*. London: Department for Education. Available at: www.gov.uk/government/publications/behaviour-in-schools--2 (Accessed: 21 March 2026).

Department for Education (2025a) *Keeping children safe in education 2025*. London: Department for Education. Available at: www.gov.uk/government/publications/keeping-children-safe-in-education--2 (Accessed: 21 March 2026).

Department for Education (2025b) *Relationships education, relationships and sex education (RSE) and health education*. London: Department for Education. Available at: www.gov.uk/government/publications/relationships-education-relationships-and-sex-education-rse-and-health-education (Accessed: 21 March 2026).

Department for Education (2026) *Working together to safeguard children 2026*. London: Department for Education. Available at: www.gov.uk/government/publications/working-together-to-safeguard-children--2 (Accessed: 21 March 2026).

Department for Education and Department of Health and Social Care (2015) *Special educational needs and disability code of practice: 0 to 25 years*. London: Department for Education and Department of Health and Social Care. Available at: www.gov.uk/government/publications/send-code-of-practice-0-to-25 (Accessed: 21 March 2026).

Eldred, E., Devries, K., Zinke-Allmang, A., Mallick, R., Mughis, W., Banks, L.M. and Bhatia, A. (2025) 'Are school-based violence prevention interventions inclusive and effective for children with disabilities? A systematic review of global evidence', *eClinicalMedicine*, 80, 103060. Available at: https://doi.org/10.1016/j.eclinm.2024.103060.

Gizzarelli, E., Burns, S. and Francis, J. (2023) 'School staff responses to student reports of bullying: A scoping review', *Health Promotion Journal of Australia*, 34(2), pp. 508–517. Available at: https://doi.org/10.1002/hpja.680.

Great Britain (2006) *Education and inspections act 2006*. London: The Stationery Office. Available at: www.legislation.gov.uk/ukpga/2006/40/contents (Accessed: 21 March 2026).

Great Britain (2010) *Equality act 2010*. London: The Stationery Office. Available at: www.legislation.gov.uk/ukpga/2010/15/contents (Accessed: 21 March 2026).

Great Britain (2014) *Children and families act 2014*. London: The Stationery Office. Available at: www.legislation.gov.uk/ukpga/2014/6/contents (Accessed: 21 March 2026).

Great Britain (2023) *Online safety act 2023*. London: The Stationery Office. Available at: www.legislation.gov.uk/ukpga/2023/50/contents (Accessed: 21 March 2026).

Grüne, B. and Willems, D. (2024) 'Help-seeking for bullying victimization among adolescents in Germany', *Child & Youth Care Forum*, 53(6), pp. 1379–1397. Available at: https://doi.org/10.1007/s10566-024-09799-4 (Accessed: 21 March 2026).

Kidwai, I. and Smith, P.K. (2024) 'A content analysis of school anti-bullying policies in England: Signs of progress', *Educational Psychology in Practice*, 40(1), pp. 1–16. Available at: https://doi.org/10.1080/02667363.2023.2250258.

Lekamge, R.B., Jain, R., Sheen, J., Solanki, P., Zhou, Y., Romero, L., Barry, M.M., Chen, L., Karim, M.N. and Ilic, D. (2025) 'Systematic review and meta-analysis of the effectiveness of whole-school interventions promoting mental health and preventing risk behaviours in adolescence', *Journal of Youth and Adolescence*, 54(2), pp. 271–289. https://doi.org/10.1007/s10964-025-02135-6.

Lester, L., Pearce, N., Waters, S., Barnes, A., Beatty, S. and Cross, D. (2017) 'Family involvement in a whole-school bullying intervention: Mothers' and fathers' communication and influence with children', *Journal of Child and Family Studies*, 26(10), pp. 2716–2727. Available at: https://doi.org/10.1007/s10826-017-0793-6.

Marchante, M., Coelho, V.A. and Romão, A.M. (2022) 'The influence of school climate in bullying and victimization behaviors during middle school transition', *Contemporary Educational Psychology*, 71, 102111. Available at: https://doi.org/10.1016/j.cedpsych.2022.102111.

Nix, T., Pendergast, D. and O'Brien, M. (2022) 'Belonging in school – The effect of teacher-student relationships: A systematic quantitative review of the literature', *Education Thinking*, 2(1), pp. 63–90.

Office of Communications (2025) *Protecting children from harms online*. London: Ofcom. Available at: www.ofcom.org.uk/online-safety/illegal-and-harmful-content/statement-protecting-children-from-harms-online (Accessed: 21 March 2026).

WHO Regional Office for Europe (2024) *A focus on adolescent peer violence and bullying in Europe, central Asia and Canada: Health behaviour in school-aged children international report from the 2021/2022 survey*. Volume 2. Copenhagen: WHO Regional Office for Europe. Available at: www.who.int/europe/publications/i/item/9789289060929 (Accessed: 21 March 2026).

Williams, S., Schneider, M., Wornell, C., Langhinrichsen-Rohling, J., Ortega, R., Ybarra, M. and Espelage, D. (2018) 'Student's perceptions of school safety: It is not just about being bullied', *Journal of School Health*, 88(1), pp. 29–37. Available at: https://doi.org/10.1111/josh.12593.

Chapter 9

When the Wounds Do Not Fade, Supporting Adult Survivors of Childhood Bullying

Abstract

Childhood bullying is often framed as a time-limited experience, yet for many adults its effects persist long after formal schooling ends. This chapter explores the enduring psychological, relational and identity-based consequences of childhood peer victimisation in adult life. It distinguishes between post-traumatic stress disorder, complex post-traumatic stress disorder and shame-based trauma responses, arguing that repeated bullying may function as chronic interpersonal trauma rather than a minor developmental challenge. Particular attention is given to identity-based bullying, including experiences linked to neurodivergence, body image, race, sexuality, disability and social difference, and to the ways these experiences shape adult self-concept and belonging. The chapter also examines the importance of meaning-making and identity reconstruction in recovery. Therapeutic pathways, including trauma-focused cognitive behavioural therapy, eye movement desensitisation and reprocessing, acceptance and commitment therapy, compassion-focused therapy, narrative work and group therapy, are considered. By reframing adult distress through a trauma-informed lens, this chapter emphasises that recovery is possible, not through forgetting the past, but through understanding it, integrating it, and rebuilding a life that is no longer governed by shame or fear.

In This Chapter

- Why the effects of childhood bullying often persist into adulthood
- The difference between post-traumatic stress disorder (PTSD), complex PTSD and shame-based trauma responses
- How bullying can shape adult identity, relationships and self-worth
- Why identity-based bullying may leave deeper and more enduring wounds
- Therapeutic pathways that support recovery, integration and rebuilding the self
- How reflective writing and meaning-making can support healing

DOI: 10.4324/9781003771777-13

A Note on Language

Throughout this chapter, person-first language is used wherever possible, including adult survivors of childhood bullying, adults affected by bullying, or adults who were bullied as children. Although terms such as victim or trauma survivor may appear in some clinical and research literature, identity labels can become fixed and reductive. The aim here is to acknowledge harm without allowing harm to become the whole story of a person's identity. Language matters in recovery. It shapes how people understand their past, their present distress and their capacity for change.

When Bullying Follows People into Adulthood

Bullying is often treated as something that belongs to childhood, a painful but temporary phase that fades with time. For many adults, however, it does not disappear. Instead, it becomes embedded in patterns of thought, feeling, bodily vigilance and self-concept. Longitudinal and qualitative evidence suggests that childhood bullying victimisation can be associated with enduring anxiety, depression, social avoidance, body-image difficulties, reduced well-being, poorer labour market outcomes and impaired adult relationships (Lidberg et al., 2022; Blanchflower and Bryson, 2024).

These adult consequences are especially important because bullying occurs during a developmental period when identity is still being formed. Repeated humiliation, exclusion, ridicule or intimidation may teach a child not only that the world is unsafe, but that they themselves are deficient, exposed or fundamentally unlikeable. In adulthood, this may appear as shame, perfectionism, fear of criticism, social camouflage or chronic anticipation of rejection. Such patterns are better understood as adaptations to repeated interpersonal threat than as evidence of personal weakness (Lidberg et al., 2022; Morgado et al., 2025).

Adult survivors do not always recognise the link between present struggles and earlier peer victimisation. They may describe burnout, social anxiety, difficulty asserting boundaries or a persistent belief that they are fundamentally unlikeable. In clinical terms, the original bullying may have ended, but the threat system has not fully stood down. The individual is still living in relation to an anticipated social danger that once had to be taken seriously.

Long-term cohort evidence suggests that the consequences of bullying are not confined to mental distress alone. Prospectively collected British birth cohort data indicate that being bullied in childhood is associated with lower subjective wellbeing across the life course, poorer labour market participation and even elevated risk of mortality before midlife, independent of other adverse childhood experiences (Blanchflower and Bryson, 2024). This matters because it resists the tendency to reduce bullying to a transient emotional injury. Its effects may become biologically, psychologically and socially embedded. The adult survivor may therefore present not only with anxiety or shame, but with disrupted employment histories, chronic stress-related symptoms, poorer physical health and reduced resilience when later life stressors arise. In this sense, bullying can be understood as a developmental stressor whose effects accumulate over time rather than disappear with age.

This broader life-course perspective helps explain why adult survivors are often confused by the depth of their own reactions. They may assume that because the bullying occurred years ago, it should no longer matter. Yet, developmental trauma does not function according to ordinary assumptions about time. When repeated humiliation, exclusion or intimidation occurs during periods of rapid emotional and neurological development, the consequences may become woven into how the person interprets relationships, risk, belonging and self-worth. The result is that adult life can become organised around old interpersonal lessons that were never consciously chosen, but were learned under duress. This is one reason bullying should be taken seriously, not only as a childhood safeguarding issue, but also as a long-term public health concern (Arseneault, 2017; Blanchflower and Bryson, 2024).

The Adult Echoes of Early Bullying

The lingering effects of childhood bullying often appear across multiple areas of adult life. Relationships may feel difficult because closeness is associated with risk. Workplaces may feel exposing because meetings, feedback and group dynamics echo earlier experiences of public scrutiny. Even positive attention can feel unsafe if visibility was once linked to ridicule.

Common adult presentations may include difficulty forming or sustaining close relationships, fear of conflict or criticism, over-apologising, perfectionism, chronic self-monitoring, avoidance of social or professional exposure, body-based shame and difficulty trusting praise. In some cases, survivors report feeling as though they suddenly become much younger in moments of stress. A minor incident in the present can reactivate an older emotional state, not because the response is irrational, but because the nervous system has learned to associate social evaluation with danger.

These reactions are often misunderstood. Adults may be told they are too sensitive, too anxious or too affected by something that happened years ago. Yet, trauma research suggests that repeated humiliation, exclusion and powerlessness can shape later emotional and relational functioning in ways that remain active well into adult life. The key point is not that every bullied child will develop long-term difficulties. It is that bullying can become developmentally significant, especially when it is chronic, identity-based or inadequately addressed.

PTSD, Complex PTSD and Shame-based Responses

A more clinically nuanced understanding is needed when considering adult survivors of childhood bullying. Not all long-term effects are captured by one diagnosis, and different survivors may present in different ways.

Post-traumatic stress disorder (PTSD) is generally associated with intrusive memories, nightmares, avoidance of reminders, hypervigilance and a persistent sense of current threat. In this formulation, the person continues to respond as though danger is still present. For some adults who experienced severe or repeated bullying, particularly involving physical violence, public humiliation or sustained intimidation, this framework may fit their presentation well.

Complex PTSD includes core trauma symptoms, but also broader disturbances in self-organisation. These include persistent emotion regulation difficulties, a deeply negative self-concept and enduring problems in relationships. This distinction is particularly relevant to survivors of childhood bullying because repeated victimisation during development does not only produce fear; it may also shape identity. A child who is repeatedly told, directly or indirectly, that they are weak, strange, disgusting or unwanted may grow into an adult whose distress is organised as much around shame and worthlessness as around fear.

Shame-based responses overlap with both PTSD and complex PTSD, but are not identical to either. Shame involves more than embarrassment. It is the painful sense that the self is fundamentally flawed, exposed or deficient. Adult survivors of bullying may carry this as an inner narrative long after the original events have passed. They may not think, 'I was harmed.' Instead, they may think, 'There is something wrong with me.' This distinction matters because treatment that addresses fear alone may not fully reach self-organisation around defectiveness and self-contempt.

For some adult survivors, the central problem is not flashbacks, but identity. They do not merely remember being bullied; they continue to live in a way that is shaped by what the bullying taught them about their value. This is why recovery often requires more than symptom management. It requires helping the person challenge meanings that were absorbed in childhood and reconstruct a self that is no longer defined by humiliation.

The distinction between PTSD, complex PTSD and shame-based distress is not merely diagnostic. It changes the kind of help survivors may need. If the presentation is viewed too narrowly through a PTSD lens, the focus may fall mainly on intrusive memories, threat responses and avoidance. These are important, but they may not capture the full burden carried by adults whose bullying was chronic, humiliating and developmentally formative. In such cases, the person may not be most distressed by flashbacks alone, but by an enduring sense of worthlessness, emotional dysregulation and persistent difficulty trusting others. This is precisely why a complex PTSD framework can be clinically helpful. It acknowledges that repeated interpersonal harm may disrupt not only the fear system, but also the developing self (Morgado et al., 2025).

Recent clinical evidence strengthens this argument. In large treatment-seeking adolescent samples from Germany, Norway and the Netherlands, bullying was a significant predictor of post-traumatic stress symptoms, even after controlling for other potentially traumatic events, age and gender, suggesting that bullying should not be dismissed as a minor or secondary stressor in trauma formulation (Sachser et al., 2025). At the same time, the symptoms most central to complex trauma often involve negative self-concept and chronic shame, features that resonate strongly with adult survivors of bullying. Li and Liang (2023) found that self-esteem partially mediated the relationship between childhood trauma and adulthood complex PTSD, with a stronger effect on disturbances in the self-organisation component than on the PTSD symptoms themselves. This is highly relevant to bullying survivors because it supports the clinical observation that the deepest injury is often not fear alone, but the internalisation of inferiority.

Shame-based responses are therefore not an optional add-on to trauma thinking. In many adult survivors, shame is the organising principle of the entire presentation. It influences how they interpret feedback, whether they believe they deserve care, how much criticism they tolerate, whether they can assert needs, and how easily they feel contaminated by exposure or failure. Some may enter therapy saying they want help with anxiety, only for the deeper formulation to reveal a shame-structured identity formed in the aftermath of years of ridicule, exclusion or social degradation. In these cases, recovery requires more than reducing arousal. It requires helping the survivor distinguish what was done to them from who they are and challenging the long-held fusion between humiliation and identity (Li and Liang, 2023; Morgado et al., 2025).

Identity-based Trauma and the Fractured Self

Bullying can be especially damaging when it is identity-based. When a child is targeted because of neurodivergence, disability, body size, race, sexuality, gender expression, class background, speech, religion or visible difference, the attack is not experienced as situational. It is experienced as an attack on the self. The message conveyed is not simply that one has done something wrong, but that one is wrong.

This kind of bullying often leaves a deeper imprint because it intersects with belonging. The child is not only being harmed by peers, but is being shown that difference can become a reason for exclusion. In adulthood, this may appear as masking, hypervigilance, internalised stigma and chronic efforts to appear acceptable. Some adults become highly skilled at adaptation and achievement, yet beneath that competence sits an unhealed fear of exposure.

Identity-based trauma can fracture self-concept in subtle but lasting ways. Survivors may distance themselves from parts of themselves that were once targeted. They may suppress their natural communication style, hide aspects of their appearance, avoid certain spaces or reject communities that remind them of their younger vulnerability. In this sense, bullying does not merely wound; it can alter the terms on which a person feels permitted to exist.

Composite Case Example: Leah's Story

Leah, a 34-year-old lecturer, sought therapy after a prolonged period of exhaustion, insomnia and escalating fear around professional visibility. She was widely regarded as capable and articulate, yet internally, she felt exposed and fraudulent. If a colleague questioned her in a meeting, she would experience an immediate surge of panic, lose her train of thought and spend days replaying the interaction. She described herself as 'still feeling like the strange girl at school'.

As therapy progressed, Leah began to speak about her childhood. Throughout secondary school, she had been bullied for being autistic, socially awkward and 'too intense'. Peers copied the way she spoke, laughed at her attempts to join conversations, and used her differences as a source of entertainment. Teachers often misread her distress as oversensitivity. Over time, Leah learned to monitor herself constantly. She studied other people carefully, rehearsed conversations in advance, and hid traits that made her feel visible. Academic excellence became both a shield and a way to earn conditional acceptance.

By adulthood, the bullying was no longer happening, yet its logic remained active. Visibility still felt dangerous. Feedback felt like humiliation. Difference felt like risk. Leah did not simply carry memories of bullying; she carried an identity built under threat.

Therapeutic work focused first on stabilisation, including sleep, grounding and recognition of bodily threat responses. From there, the work moved towards shame and meaning. Leah began to recognise that many of her beliefs about herself had not emerged from truth, but from repeated social injury. She also joined a neurodivergent peer support group, where, for the first time, she experienced recognition rather than judgement. That experience mattered profoundly. It helped shift her understanding of herself from defective to different. Recovery did not involve erasing the past. It involved reclaiming the right to exist without constant camouflage.

Meaning-making and Identity Reconstruction

One of the most important tasks in adult recovery is meaning-making. Bullying does not only hurt in the moment; it shapes what the survivor comes to believe about their self, others and the world. It may lead to beliefs such as 'I am unsafe when noticed', 'People will reject the real me', or 'If I make a mistake, I will be humiliated'. These meanings can persist long after the original context has changed.

Meaning-making is not about finding a positive lesson in suffering. It is about understanding what happened accurately enough that the survivor no longer interprets their adaptation as personal failure. This can be profoundly relieving. When a person begins to see that their anxiety, perfectionism or withdrawal developed in response to repeated social threat, self-blame can begin to loosen.

Closely linked to meaning-making is identity reconstruction. Many adult survivors are still living from identities formed under siege. They know how to survive, but not always how to feel safe. They know how to minimise themselves, but not how to inhabit themselves fully. Recovery therefore involves more than reducing symptoms. It involves asking who the person is beneath the strategies that once kept them alive socially and emotionally.

This process may include grief. Survivors may mourn the confidence, spontaneity or developmental ease that bullying interrupted. It may include anger, particularly where adults failed to protect them. It may also include compassion for the younger self who adapted as best they could. Identity reconstruction is slow, because it is not cosmetic. It is the rebuilding of a self that was shaped in relation to chronic exposure, shame or exclusion.

Meaning-making also has an interpersonal dimension. Adult survivors are often not only trying to understand what happened, but why no one stopped it, why it lasted so long, and what it came to mean about their place in the world. For some, the most injurious aspect of bullying was not the aggressor's behaviour alone, but the silence of peers, staff or family members who failed to intervene. This failure can become part of the trauma narrative, reinforcing beliefs that one is unworthy of protection or that suffering will not be taken seriously. In adulthood, this may shape help-seeking, disclosure and the ability to trust therapeutic relationships. Oexle et al. (2020) found that bullying victimisation was linked to later mental health service use, with self-labelling playing a mediating role. This suggests that the survivor's understanding of themselves, whether as damaged, ill, weak or harmed, may influence both distress and pathways into support.

Identity reconstruction therefore involves more than developing confidence. It involves the careful rebuilding of moral and relational meaning. Survivors may need to grieve the fact that they were not defended, name the injustice of what happened, and re-evaluate assumptions that grew around this neglect. Some begin adult life believing they must tolerate mistreatment because that is simply how relationships work. Others assume that being disliked or excluded is an inevitable response to their authentic self. Recovery requires these assumptions to be examined and, where possible, revised. It also involves creating a self-story large enough to contain both vulnerability and strength. The adult survivor is not only the child who was bullied. They are also the person who endured, adapted and now has the possibility of living differently. That shift from humiliation-based identity to authored identity is often one of the most important outcomes of healing (Oexle et al., 2020; Lidberg et al., 2022).

Revictimisation, Intimate Partner Violence and Adult Relationships

For some adult survivors, the legacy of childhood bullying may extend beyond anxiety, shame and social withdrawal into later patterns of revictimisation. The current evidence base does not justify claiming that childhood bullying straightforwardly causes domestic abuse in adulthood. However, it does suggest that bullying victimisation may increase later vulnerability to interpersonal victimisation, including abuse and control within intimate relationships (Adhia et al., 2019; Strøm et al., 2025).

This distinction matters. A deterministic statement would overreach the evidence and risk misrepresenting survivors' futures as fixed. A trauma-informed interpretation is more accurate. Repeated bullying may shape how safety, conflict, rejection and power are understood in later relationships. Survivors who have grown up under conditions of humiliation, exclusion or chronic criticism may enter adulthood with impaired self-worth, heightened tolerance of mistreatment, difficulty identifying coercive behaviour early or a strong drive to appease others in order to avoid abandonment or further attack. These are not character flaws; they are adaptations to interpersonal threat (Swee et al., 2024; Morgado et al., 2025).

The strongest direct evidence comes from studies of revictimisation. In a national Norwegian study of adults, one in five participants reported childhood bullying victimisation, and approximately half of these individuals reported victimisation again in adulthood, including controlling behaviour from a partner, rape or severe physical violence. Even after adjustment for sociodemographic factors, childhood bullying remained associated with significantly higher odds of adulthood victimisation, with an adjusted odds ratio of 1.52 compared with those who reported neither childhood bullying nor childhood violence (Strøm et al., 2025).

Prospective evidence points in the same direction. In a US cohort study, participants who reported being bullied more than twice in adolescence were at elevated risk of later intimate partner violence victimisation in young adulthood, even after adjustment for bullying perpetration, childhood abuse history and other covariates. The authors concluded that modes of interaction learned or normalised in peer relationships may carry forward into dating relationships, increasing later vulnerability to abuse (Adhia et al., 2019).

These findings do not mean that survivors of bullying are destined to experience domestic abuse. Many do not. However, they do suggest that clinicians and support workers should remain alert to the possibility that unresolved bullying trauma may contribute to later relational risk. This may be especially true where bullying has become internalised as shame, worthlessness or a belief that poor treatment must be tolerated in order to maintain connection. Adult survivors may therefore need help not only with processing past peer victimisation, but also with recognising coercion, strengthening boundaries, rebuilding relational trust and developing a self-concept that is no longer organised around fear and submission (Lidberg et al., 2022; Morgado et al., 2025).

In this sense, bullying may be understood not simply as a historical school experience, but as a developmental injury that can shape later expectations of intimacy, power and safety. Where this occurs, recovery requires more than symptom reduction. It requires rebuilding the survivor's sense of what respectful relationships feel like, and what they are entitled to expect from others.

Therapeutic Pathways for Healing

There is no single treatment pathway for adult survivors of childhood bullying, and therapy is most effective when it is guided by formulation rather than applied mechanically. Some survivors present with more classic trauma symptoms, such as intrusive recollections, physiological reactivity and avoidance. Others present with chronic shame, fractured identity and longstanding relational difficulty. Many present with all these symptoms. This means that the therapeutic task is not simply to choose a named intervention, but to understand which aspects of the bullying legacy are most active in the present.

Trauma-focused cognitive behavioural therapy (TF-CBT) and eye movement desensitisation and reprocessing (EMDR) remain important where the adult survivor's presentation is strongly organised around intrusive memories, avoidance and bodily threat responses. These approaches may help reduce the intensity of trauma-linked reactivity and challenge fixed cognitions such as 'I am powerless' or 'I am never safe'. They can be especially useful where specific episodes of bullying remain vivid and emotionally overwhelming. However, adult survivors of bullying often need treatment that goes beyond fear-based trauma processing, particularly where the injury has become embedded in self-worth, relational expectations or chronic self-criticism.

Acceptance and commitment therapy (ACT) offers one useful route here. ACT is especially relevant when the survivor's life has become narrowed by avoidance, shame or fusion with painful internal experiences. Rather than trying to eliminate distressing thoughts, ACT helps individuals notice them differently, create distance from them, and move towards values-based action, even when discomfort remains present. For adult survivors of bullying, this can support a shift away from lives organised around concealment, appeasement or fear of judgment. A recent systematic review and meta-analysis found a moderate and statistically significant overall effect of ACT on reducing trauma-related symptoms in adults, suggesting it is a credible trauma-informed option, even though the evidence base is broader than bullying-specific populations (Rowe-Johnson et al., 2025). Its emphasis on psychological flexibility is particularly compatible with survivors who remain trapped in rigid self-protective patterns long after the original threat has ended.

Compassion-focused therapy (CFT) may be even more directly relevant where shame and self-criticism sit at the centre of the presentation. Repeated bullying often leaves behind an internal persecutor, a voice that continues the logic of humiliation after the original aggressors have gone. CFT was developed specifically to address shame and self-criticism, making it highly applicable to bullying survivors whose inner world remains organised around defectiveness and self-attack. Swee et al. (2024) argue that CFT may be particularly suitable for ICD-11 complex PTSD because it targets disturbances in self-organisation, especially negative self-concept, emotion regulation difficulties and relational mistrust. These are all features commonly seen in adults whose bullying histories were prolonged, identity-based or marked by repeated public humiliation.

Importantly, support for CFT is no longer only theoretical. In a randomised controlled trial of adults meeting ICD-11 criteria for complex PTSD, Ríos-Mercado et al. (2025) found that compassion-focused therapy produced significant reductions in post-traumatic symptoms, shame, self-criticism, depression, anxiety, stress and dissociation. It also increased self-compassion and self-soothing, with higher completion rates than prolonged exposure. This is particularly important for bullying survivors, many of whom may find directly exposure-oriented work difficult if warmth, care or self-kindness have historically felt unsafe. In such cases, building internal safeness may be a necessary foundation for deeper trauma work.

Narrative approaches also deserve emphasis. Bullying often compresses a person's identity into the meanings imposed by others. The survivor may have spent years being interpreted through the bully's lens as weak, strange, unattractive, excessive, inferior or fundamentally unlikeable. Narrative therapy and other meaning-focused approaches can help externalise the bullying, examine the beliefs it generated, and support re-authoring of the self. This does not mean imposing a falsely triumphant story. It means helping the survivor build a more accurate and compassionate narrative, one in which the experience is acknowledged without being allowed total authority over identity.

Group therapy and peer support can also play a significant role, although this part of the evidence base is less specific to bullying survivors than the literature on trauma more broadly. Even so, the rationale is compelling. Bullying is a relational injury, so some aspects of healing may occur most meaningfully in the presence of others. Carefully facilitated groups may offer validation, reduce shame, challenge distorted self-perceptions and provide a corrective experience of being seen without ridicule. For survivors of identity-based bullying, groups can be especially reparative because they restore the possibility of belonging where exclusion once dominated. This is often the beginning of relational healing, not because the past is erased, but because the person has a new experience against which to measure it.

In practice, many survivors benefit from an integrative approach. They may need stabilisation and psychoeducation first, followed by trauma processing, compassion-based work, and later relational or identity reconstruction. Some may require work on boundaries and coercion awareness, particularly if revictimisation or abusive relationships have become part of the adult pattern. Others may need help with embodiment, reclaiming their voice or reducing perfectionistic over-functioning. The most effective treatment is therefore not the most fashionable or intensive one, but the one that best matches the survivor's actual formulation. The central question is not simply 'What therapy works for bullying?', but 'What aspects of this person's adult life are still being governed by the bullying, and what kind of therapeutic work will help loosen that hold?' (Swee et al., 2024; Ríos-Mercado et al., 2025; Rowe-Johnson et al., 2025).

Reflective Writing and Healing

Writing can help survivors process experiences that were never fully named or understood at the time. It can also help separate the voice of the bully from the voice of the self. The aim is not to reopen wounds carelessly, but to create language for what has previously been carried in silence.

The following prompts may support reflection and therapeutic exploration:

- What did I come to believe about myself because of the bullying, and whose voice do those beliefs belong to?
- When do I feel most pulled back into my younger bullied self, and what helps me return to the present?
- What parts of myself did I learn to hide in order to stay safe?
- What would I say now to the younger version of me who believed the bullying was their fault?
- What strengths helped me survive, and which of those still serve me today?
- What would it mean to build an identity that is not organised around fear, shame or concealment?

One useful exercise is to write two letters. In the first, the younger self describes what it was like to be bullied. In the second, the adult self responds with witness, protection and compassion. This can help move the survivor from silent endurance towards active self-repair.

Conclusion

For many adults, childhood bullying is not over simply because it happened years ago. Its effects may persist in the body, in relationships, in self-worth, and in the narratives people hold about who they are allowed to be. Some survivors live with symptoms that resemble PTSD. Others present more clearly with complex PTSD or shame-based patterns of distress. Many carry elements of all three.

A trauma-informed understanding is therefore essential. It allows adult struggles to be interpreted not as overreaction or weakness, but as meaningful responses to repeated social harm during development. Recovery is possible, but it rarely comes from minimising what happened. It comes from naming it accurately, understanding its impact, processing its emotional residue, and rebuilding an identity that is no longer controlled by fear or humiliation.

The wounds may not simply fade with time. But with understanding, support and the right therapeutic conditions, they do not have to define the whole of a person's life.

Key Takeaways

- Childhood bullying can shape adult identity, relationships and nervous system responses long after school ends
- PTSD, complex PTSD and shame-based responses overlap, but they are not the same and require careful clinical understanding
- Identity-based bullying often leaves deeper wounds because it targets belonging, as well as safety
- Recovery involves more than symptom reduction, it also involves meaning-making and identity reconstruction
- Therapeutic approaches such as TF-CBT, EMDR, ACT, compassion-focused therapy, narrative work and group support may all play a role
- Healing is possible when adult survivors are helped to understand their distress as adaptation rather than personal failure

References

Adhia, A., Gordon, A.R., Roberts, A.L., Fitzmaurice, G.M., Hemenway, D. and Austin, S.B. (2019) 'Longitudinal associations between bullying and intimate partner violence among adolescents and young adults', *Violence and Victims*, 34(6), pp. 1011–1029. https://doi.org/10.1891/0886-6708.VV-D-18-00135

Arseneault, L. (2017) 'The long-term impact of bullying victimization on mental health', *World Psychiatry*, 16(1), pp. 27–28.

Blanchflower, D.G. and Bryson, A. (2024) 'The adult consequences of being bullied in childhood', *Social Science & Medicine*, 345, 116690. https://doi.org/10.1016/j.socscimed.2024.116690.

Li, Y. and Liang, Y. (2023) 'The effect of childhood trauma on complex posttraumatic stress disorder: The role of self-esteem', *European Journal of Psychotraumatology*, 14(2), 2272478. https://doi.org/10.1080/20008066.2023.2272478.

Lidberg, J., Berne, S. and Frisén, A. (2022) 'Challenges in emerging adulthood related to the impact of childhood bullying victimization', *Emerging Adulthood*, 11(2), pp. 346–364. https://doi.org/10.1177/21676968211051475.

Morgado, D., Correia-Santos, P., Pinto, R. and Maia, Â. (2025) 'Bullying victimization and complex trauma: A systematic review of CPTSD and DTD symptoms', *Trauma, Violence, & Abuse*, [online], pp. 1–16. https://doi.org/10.1177/15248380251401923.

Oexle, N., Ribeiro, W., Fisher, H.L., Gronholm, P.C., Laurens, K.R., Pan, P., Owens, S., Romeo, R., Rüsch, N. and Evans-Lacko, S. (2020) 'Childhood bullying victimization, self-labelling, and help-seeking for mental health problems', *Social Psychiatry and Psychiatric Epidemiology*, 55, pp. 81–88. https://doi.org/10.1007/s00127-019-01743-5.

Ríos-Mercado, S.P., Tena-Suck, A., Lucio y Gómez-Maqueo, M.E., Villafuerte-Montiel, A.L. and Fuentes-Balderrama, J. (2025) 'Compassion focused therapy for complex posttraumatic stress disorder: A randomized controlled trial', *Journal of Psychopathology and Clinical Psychology / Revista de Psicopatología y Psicología Clínica*, 30(3), pp. 217–231. https://doi.org/10.5944/rppc.44336.

Rowe-Johnson, M.K., Browning, B. and Scott, B. (2025) 'Effects of acceptance and commitment therapy on trauma-related symptoms: A systematic review and meta-analysis', *Psychological Trauma: Theory, Research, Practice, and Policy*, 17(3), pp. 668–675. https://doi.org/10.1037/tra0001785.

Sachser, C., Kooij, L.H., Keller, J., Eilers, R., Jensen, T.K., Lindauer, R.J.L., Ormhaug, S.M., Pfeiffer, E., Rosner, R., Solheim Skar, A.-M. and Birkeland, M.S. (2025) 'Understanding bullying as a significant predictor of posttraumatic stress symptoms in adolescents: Insights from clinical samples in Norway, The Netherlands and Germany', *European Journal of Psychotraumatology*, 16(1), 2589566. https://doi.org/10.1080/20008066.2025.2589566.

Strøm, I.F., Aakvaag, H.F., Nissen, A., Skauge, A.D., Seifert, L.C., Nielsen, M.B. and Dale, M.T.G. (2025) 'The prevalence of childhood bullying and violence victimization and subsequent risk of adult revictimization in the Norwegian population: A cross-sectional study', *Journal of Traumatic Stress*, 38(3), pp. 458–469. https://doi.org/10.1002/jts.23145.

Swee, M.B., Corman, A.G., Margolis, J.M. and Dick, A.M. (2024) 'Compassion-focused therapy for the treatment of ICD-11-defined complex posttraumatic stress disorder', *American Journal of Psychotherapy*, 77(3), pp. 135–140. https://doi.org/10.1176/appi.psychotherapy.20230019.

Conclusion

A Call to Action

Abstract

This conclusion brings together the central argument of the book: bullying is not a harmless childhood experience, but a serious developmental, emotional and public health issue. Drawing together the neuroscience, trauma research, educational evidence and lived experiences explored throughout the book, it shows how bullying can shape stress responses, identity, self-worth and mental health across the life course. It also reinforces the need to move beyond individual blame and towards trauma-informed, relational and systemic responses. Parents, educators, health professionals and policymakers all play a role in recognising the hidden impact of bullying, responding early, and creating environments where children and young people feel safe, believed and supported. The chapter ends by emphasising hope, recovery and prevention, arguing that when adults understand the developing brain, they are better equipped to protect children from harm and support healing after bullying.

Why This Book Matters

The central argument of this book is simple, but its implications are far-reaching. Bullying should no longer be dismissed as a minor behavioural problem, a normal part of growing up, or an unfortunate but inevitable feature of school life. The research reviewed across these chapters suggests something more serious. Repeated peer victimisation can disrupt a child's sense of safety, belonging, trust and self-worth. It can affect learning, attendance, emotional regulation, peer relationships and, for some children, longer-term mental health and social functioning (Wolke and Lereya, 2015; Arseneault, 2018). When these harms are widespread, preventable and unequally distributed, they become more than an individual problem. They become a public health concern.

That framing matters because it shifts the question. Instead of asking only how to stop a single incident, we begin to ask what conditions make bullying

DOI: 10.4324/9781003771777-14

more likely, what protects children from harm, and how systems respond before distress becomes entrenched. Public health approaches focus on prevention, early recognition, risk reduction, protective environments and coordinated support. They also recognise that harms are patterned socially rather than distributed evenly. Children who are already marginalised, including disabled children, neurodivergent children and children targeted because of race, sexuality, gender expression, poverty, appearance or perceived difference, may face both greater exposure and greater consequences. In that sense, bullying is not only a developmental issue. It is also an issue of inequality, safeguarding and social justice (UNESCO, 2019; WHO Regional Office for Europe, 2024).

Why Nuance Matters

At the same time, this book has argued consistently for nuance. Not all bullying leads to trauma. Not every child who is bullied will go on to develop a mental health disorder. Some children recover relatively quickly once the bullying stops and meaningful protection is put in place. Others show distress in one domain, but not in another. Some appear outwardly calm, while carrying significant internal strain. These differences matter. They remind us that we are dealing with probabilities, not certainties; risk, not destiny; and human beings, not fixed categories. The more accurate position is that bullying can be profoundly harmful, sometimes traumatising, often underestimated, and always deserving of serious adult attention.

This nuanced position is especially important when discussing the brain. Across the book, the aim has not been to claim that bullying damages every child in the same way or that neuroscience can explain the whole of human suffering. Rather, the evidence suggests that chronic peer threat can place sustained pressure on stress systems and on the developmental processes that support learning, attention, emotion regulation and social confidence. For some children, particularly when bullying is repeated, humiliating, inescapable or identity-based, the body and brain may adapt to threat in ways that persist beyond the original context. Hypervigilance, shutdown, avoidance, irritability, poor sleep, concentration difficulties and negative self-beliefs are often understandable adaptations to prolonged social danger. Yet adaptation is not the same as permanence. Recovery remains possible, especially when safety, predictable support and trusted relationships are restored.

It is often said that children are resilient. There is some truth in this, because many children do recover and adapt following adversity. However, resilience is not an automatic trait, nor is it evidence that harm was insignificant. Resilience is better understood as a dynamic process, shaped by the interaction between the child and the protective factors around them, especially stable supportive relationships, opportunities to build coping and self-regulation skills, and safe, predictable environments (Masten and Barnes, 2018; Center on the Developing Child at Harvard University, 2015). Evidence from a systematic review also suggests that resilient outcomes in children exposed to social adversity are associated with protective factors across the child, family, school and community, rather than with individual strength alone (Gartland et al., 2019). For that reason, the phrase 'children are resilient' should never be used to minimise bullying or justify adult inaction. A more accurate position is that children may show resilience when adults, services and systems create the conditions that make recovery possible (Mesman et al., 2021).

Recovery is Possible, but Prevention Matters Most

This is why the book has placed equal weight on harm and recovery. It is not enough to document what bullying can do; we must also be clear about what helps. Children recover best when adults respond early, respond consistently and respond relationally. Safety cannot be reduced to a policy statement. It has to be felt in the child's body, in the classroom, in friendships, online and at home. A child who has been repeatedly humiliated does not simply need to be told that the bullying has stopped. They need evidence, over time, that adults can be trusted, that routines are predictable, and that they are more than what happened to them. Recovery often begins with containment and protection, but it grows through connection, agency and the gradual rebuilding of belonging.

The evidence for prevention points in the same direction. Bullying is less likely to thrive in environments where adults are attentive, school climate is consistent, peer norms do not reward cruelty, and inclusion is actively practised rather than merely stated. Whole-school approaches are not perfect, and effects are not uniform across all contexts, but they offer one of the strongest available directions of travel. The recent UK trial of KiVa, for example, found reductions in victimisation and improvements in empathy, while also reminding us that implementation quality matters as much as programme design (Bowes et al., 2024). Children are not protected by slogans. They are protected by sustained systems, trained adults, clear pathways and cultures in which unkindness is challenged early and belonging is taken seriously.

A Shared Responsibility

For parents, the task is rarely to solve everything at once. It is to notice changes, create emotional safety, listen without minimising, and stay steady enough for the child to borrow calm. Many children do not disclose bullying directly. They show it through school refusal, disrupted sleep, irritability, sudden withdrawal or a shrinking world. Parents are often the first to see these changes, and their response can shape whether shame deepens or begins to loosen. Believing the child does not mean assuming every detail is already clear. It means taking their distress seriously, asking careful questions, documenting concerns and working persistently with the school or wider services when needed.

For teachers and school leaders, the message is equally clear. Bullying cannot be treated as an isolated behavioural issue detached from classroom climate, peer dynamics, safeguarding, attendance and inclusion. Children who are distressed do not always present as vulnerable. Some become quiet and compliant; some become angry, disruptive, or avoidant. A trauma-informed school response is therefore not a soft alternative to discipline. It is a more accurate and effective way of understanding behaviour, context and recovery. Staff need the confidence to distinguish conflict from bullying, to recognise identity-based harms, to intervene in group processes rather than waiting for repeated complaints, and to follow through long after the initial disclosure.

For health and mental health professionals, one of the most important lessons is that bullying should not sit at the margins of assessment. Peer relationships are central to development, and repeated victimisation may be clinically relevant in presentations involving anxiety, depression, self-harm, trauma symptoms, emotional dysregulation, school avoidance, eating difficulties, somatic complaints or social withdrawal. Asking directly, but sensitively, about bullying and exclusion should be part of good developmental enquiry. Equally important is the need for formulation rather than over-simplification. Some children need practical advocacy and a safer environment. Some need trauma-focused intervention. Some need work that addresses shame, identity and meaning-making.

For policymakers, the call to action is urgent because policy shapes the conditions in which all other responses occur. If bullying remains dispersed across behaviour, safeguarding, equality, special education needs and disabilities, attendance and online safety agendas without clear coordination, children will continue to fall between systems. Policy must do more than require schools to have an anti-bullying statement. It must support training, accountability, implementation and inter-agency pathways. It must recognise that cyberbullying extends harm beyond the school gate and that prevention depends partly on digital regulation, as well as school practice. A serious policy response measures more than incident counts. It asks whether children feel safe, whether they trust adults, whether they seek help, and whether vulnerable groups are protected in practice rather than on paper (WHO Regional Office for Europe, 2024).

Across the Lifespan

This book has also argued that the impact of bullying does not necessarily end when school does. For some adults, childhood bullying remains present in the form of avoidance, shame, mistrust, perfectionism, relational fear or a persistent sense of social unsafety. This does not mean that adult survivors are permanently defined by childhood victimisation. It means that repeated interpersonal humiliation can become woven into identity in ways that take time to name and undo. Adult distress linked to childhood bullying is neither trivial nor inexplicable. It deserves understanding and, where appropriate, clinical care.

If there is one lesson that should remain after the last page of this book, it is that listening to children is not sentimental, it is foundational. Adults often ask children to report bullying, but not all children believe that reporting will change anything. Some have already learned that disclosure leads to minimisation, delay, retaliation or paperwork without protection. Rebuilding trust therefore requires more than encouraging children to speak. It requires adults to respond in ways that are timely, coherent, and visible. The real test of an anti-bullying response is not how strong it sounds in policy language, but whether children experience it as credible.

What You Can Do Today

Parents can begin with a daily emotional check-in, using language that makes feelings easier to name. Teachers can introduce brief, predictable routines that help pupils regulate, and can use simple wellbeing check-ins to identify children whose distress is otherwise hidden. Health professionals can ask directly about friendships, exclusion and bullying when assessing mood, anxiety, risk or school avoidance. School leaders can review whether current procedures merely record incidents or actually produce safety. Policymakers can ask whether the existing framework is coherent enough for families and practitioners to navigate without delay.

Final Reflection

Bullying is preventable, even if it cannot be eliminated completely from every setting. Its harms can be reduced. Recovery can be supported. Systems can improve. That is the note on which this book should end. Not false reassurance, and not despair, but responsibility. Children need adults who understand the difference between conflict and cruelty, who recognise that repeated humiliation can shape development, and who are willing to act before harm becomes part of a child's identity. We owe children more than awareness. We owe them protection, dignity and the chance to grow in environments where safety and belonging are ordinary rather than exceptional.

References

Arseneault, L. (2018) 'Annual research review: The persistent and pervasive impact of being bullied in childhood and adolescence: Implications for policy and practice', *Journal of Child Psychology and Psychiatry*, 59(4), pp. 405–421. doi:10.1111/jcpp.12841.

Bowes, L., Babu, M., Badger, J.R., Broome, M.R., Cannings-John, R., Clarkson, S., Coulman, E., Edwards, R.T., Ford, T., Hastings, R.P., Hayes, R., Lugg-Widger, F., Owen-Jones, E., Patterson, P., Segrott, J., Sydenham, M., Townson, J., Watkins, R.C., Whiteley, H., Williams, M.E., the Stand Together Team and Hutchings, J. (2024) The effects and costs of an anti-bullying program (KiVa) in UK primary schools: A multicenter cluster randomized controlled trial. *Psychological Medicine*, 54(15), pp. 4362–4373. https://doi.org/10.1017/S0033291724002666.

Center on the Developing Child at Harvard University (2015) *InBrief: The science of resilience*. Available at: https://developingchild.harvard.edu/resources/inbriefs/inbrief-the-science-of-resilience/ (Accessed: 6 April 2026).

Gartland, D., Riggs, E., Muyeen, S., Giallo, R., Afifi, T.O., MacMillan, H., Herrman, H., Bulford, E. and Brown, S.J. (2019) 'What factors are associated with resilient outcomes in children exposed to social adversity? A systematic review', *BMJ Open*, 9(4), e024870. https://doi.org/10.1136/bmjopen-2018-024870.

Masten, A.S. and Barnes, A.J. (2018) 'Resilience in children: Developmental perspectives', *Children*, 5(7), p. 98. https://doi.org/10.3390/children5070098.

Mesman, E., Vreeker, A. and Hillegers, M. (2021) 'Resilience and mental health in children and adolescents: An update of the recent literature and future directions', *Current Opinion in Psychiatry*, 34(6), pp. 586–592. https://doi.org/10.1097/YCO.0000000000000741.

UNESCO (2019) *Behind the numbers: Ending school violence and bullying*. Paris: UNESCO.

WHO Regional Office for Europe (2024) *A focus on adolescent peer violence and bullying in Europe, central Asia and Canada: Health behaviour in school-aged children international report from the 2021/2022 survey*. Volume 2. Copenhagen: WHO Regional Office for Europe.

Wolke, D. and Lereya, S.T. (2015) 'Long-term effects of bullying', *Archives of Disease in Childhood*, 100(9), pp. 879–885.

Index

Note: Page numbers in **bold** and *italics* represents tables and figures, respectively.

For Product Safety Concerns and Information please contact our EU representative GPSR@taylorandfrancis.com Taylor & Francis Verlag GmbH, Kaufingerstraße 24, 80331 München, Germany